Quick and easy ketogenic cooking book

The ketogenic diet is a popular low carb diet that pushes the body to produce ketones used by the liver as energy. Naturally, the body produces insulin and glucose when you eat foods high in carbohydrates. The glucose is used as energy and insulin processes the glucose in the blood and takes it around the body.

When this happens, fats that aren't needed by the body are stored. When the carbohydrate intake is lowered, the body enters into ketosis.

Ketosis is a natural process the body initiates to help us survive when food intake is low. During this state, we produce ketones, which are produced from the breakdown of fats in the liver.

The main goal of a keto diet is to push the body into the metabolic state of ketosis. Regular starvation of calories cannot trigger this effect, only starvation of carbohydrates can do it. The body adapts to whatever is put in it. When it is overloaded with fats, and the carbohydrates are removed, it starts to use ketones as energy. Having optimal ketones levels have been proven to offer lots of weight loss, health, mental, physical and performance benefits.

This book will provide a comprehensive list of ketogenic diet recipes as well as methods to prepare them to ease your journey into a healthier life. Keto diets do not need to be bland and boring; you will find some tasty meals to try out at home. They are also very easy to make. Sit back and enjoy this guide.

Оглавление

Breakfast Recipes 7
    Avocado Toad in the Hole 8
    Bacon, Egg and Cheese Cups: 9
    Brie and Apple Crepes: 11
    Steak and Eggs: 13
    Basic Oopsie Rolls 14
    Mini Egg Quiches 15
    Scrambled Eggs 16
    Low Carb and Paleo Cereal 17
    Blueberry Coconut Porridge 18
    Fat-Burning Vanilla Smoothie 19

Salad recipes 20
    Strawberry Cheesecake Salad 21
    Curried Cabbage Coconut Salad 22
    Coconut & Turmeric Chia Pudding 23
    Halloumi Stuffed Peppers 24
    Feta Lemon Coleslaw 25
    Greek Goddess Kale Salad 26
    Summer Confetti Salad 28
    Amish Broccoli Cauliflower Salad 29
    Cucumber Salad (Thai) 30
    Grilled Chicken Breast Salad 32

Soup recipes 33
    Ham And Green Bean Soup 34
    Cauliflower and ham soup 35
    Moqueca De Camaroes 36

- Roasted Broccoli & Cheddar Soup 37
- Avgolemono soup 38
- Jalapeno popper soup 39
- Mulligatawny Soup 40
- Pumpkin Chipotle Soup 41
- Cream of tomato soup 42
- Greens Cream Soup 43

Lunch recipes 44
- Salami rollups 45
- Protein roll 46
- Avocado burrata and cheese chips 47
- Cheese and ham toasted sandwich 48
- Avocado salad, prawns, and toasted bread 49
- Bacon whiskey caramelized onions 50
- Tamari Marinated Steak Salad 51
- Chicken Bites 52
- Mustard Sardines Salad 53
- Mini Zucchini Avocado Burgers 54

Dessert recipes 56
- Coconut Oil Candies 57
- Chocolate Ice Cream 58
- Instant Avocado Vanilla Pudding 59
- Sugar-free Lemon Curd 60
- Lemon cloud pie 61
- Fresh Fruit Tart 62
- No-Bake Rhubarb Crisp 63
- Strawberry Cream Pie 64
- Cheesecake Salad 65
- Cherry Chocolate Cheesecake 66

Meat recipes 67
- Corned beef hash 68
- Low Carb Beef Burritos 69
- Bacon and Beef Roll-Ups 70
- Malaysian Beef Curry 71
- Homemade Beef Jerky 73
- Fish Curry with Coconut and Spinach 74
- Meatloaf Cupcakes 75
- Parmesan-Encrusted Halibut 76
- Lamb meatballs 77
- Keto teriyaki beef 79
- Keto buffalo chicken soup 81
- Sriracha Ranch Chicken 82
- Taco Lime Grilled Chicken 84
- Chicken and Avocado Burritos 85
- Chicken in Creamy Parmesan with Sundried Tomato Sauce 86

Dinner recipes 88
- Spaghetti A la Carbonara 89
- One Pot Shrimp Alfredo 90
- Keto Cordon Bleu 92
- Savory Italian Egg Bake 94
- Keto Sushi 96
- Keto Hot Chili Soup 98
- Keto Pumpkin Carbonara 100
- Coconut Curry Chicken Tenders 102
- Chicken Pad Thai 104
- Low-Carb Chicken Curry 106
- Salmon with Tarragon Dill Cream Sauce 108
- Orange and Sage Glazed Duck Breast 110

    Perfect Ribeye Steak 111

    Roasted Red Bell Pepper and Cauliflower Soup 112

    Bacon Cheeseburger Soup 114

Snacks recipe 116

    Almonds Italiano 117

    Tortilla Chips 118

    Almond Flour Crisps 119

    Microwave Flax Crackers 120

    WPI Crackers 121

    Chewy Peanut Butter Candy 122

    Chocolate Almond Bar 123

    Chocolate Coconut Bark 124

    Coconut Fudge 125

    Whey Protein Not Cake 126

Sauce recipes 127

    Brown Butter Cream sauce 128

    Keto Spicy BBQ Sauce 129

    Cocktail Sauce 131

    Enchilada Sauce 132

    Sweet Soy Sauce 133

    Grocery list 134

Diet plan 139

Why you should keep track of your figure and health 140

THANK YOU FOR BUYING MY BOOK!

Just take your gift from me

http://www.bestsellers.pp.ua/robertstill/

Thank You!

Robert Still

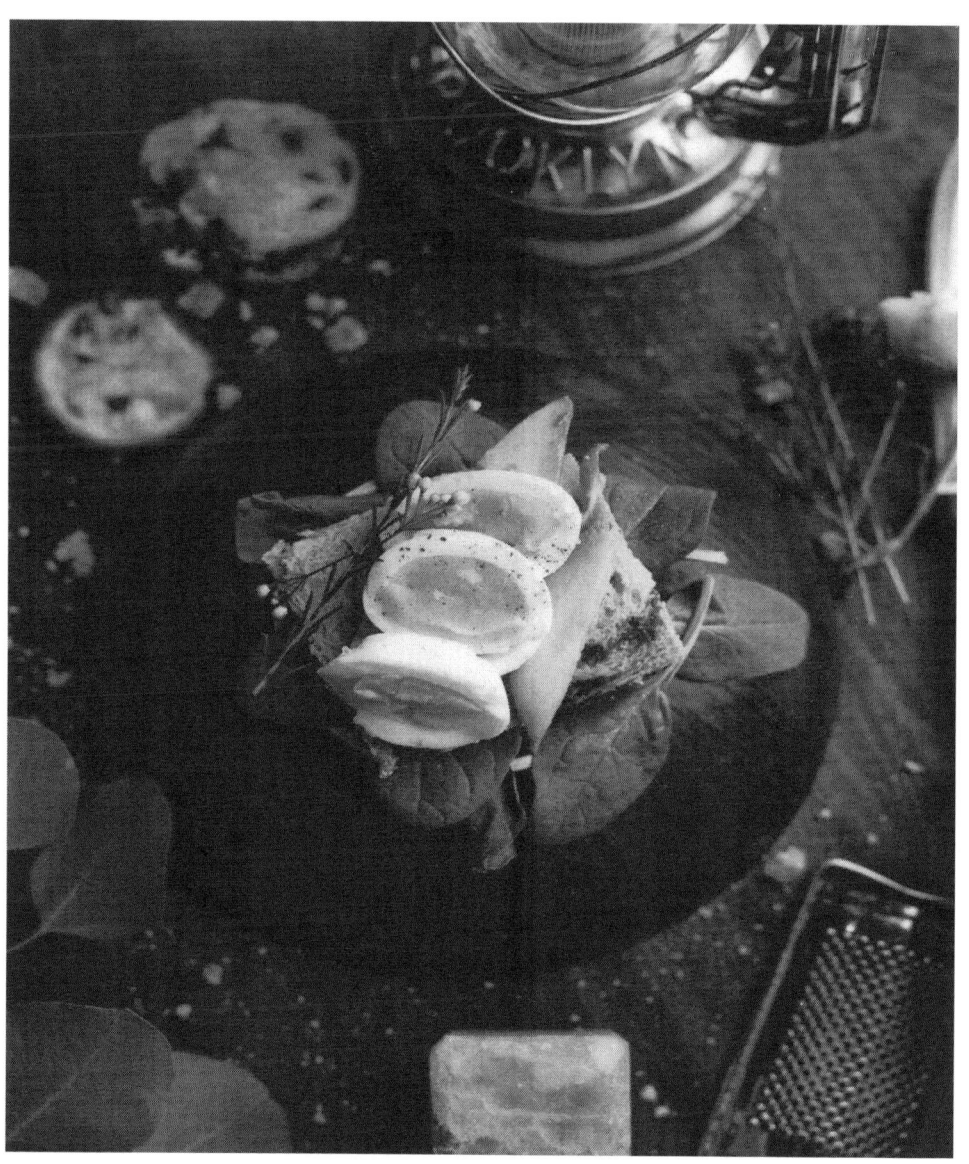

Breakfast Recipes

Avocado Toad in the Hole:

Makes: 6 servings

Serving size: 3 avocados

Calories: 261 Calories

Preparation time: 10 minutes

Nutritional information:

Fat   20g

Protein   14g

Carbohydrate   3g

Fiber   5g

Ingredients:

1. 3 medium avocados
2. 6 medium eggs
3. 1/2 tsp sea salt
4. 1 tsp garlic powder
5. 1/4 cup Parmesan cheese
6. 1/4 tsp black pepper

Instructions

1. Preheat your oven to 350°F, cut three avocados in half, and remove the pits.
2. Put the avocado halves in a muffin tin.
3. Sprinkle sea salt, garlic powder, and black pepper on the halves.
4. Crack one egg into the avocado and sprinkle cheese over the eggs.
5. Place in the oven for 12-15 minutes.

Bacon, Egg and Cheese Cups:

Makes: 12 servings
Serving size: 1 cup
Calories: 101
Preparation time: 15 minutes

Nutritional information:
Fat   7g
Protein   8g
Carbohydrates   1g

Ingredients:
1. 12 large eggs
2. 12 bacon strips
3. 1/2 cup frozen spinach
4. Salt and pepper
5. 1/3 cup cheddar cheese

Instructions:
1. Preheat your oven to 400°F.
2. Fry the slices of bacon in a pan.
3. Grease your muffin pan generously using olive oil or coconut oil and line each cup with a slice of bacon.

4. Push the slice down so that it will stick up on any side.
5. Crack and beat the eggs in a large bowl.
6. Stir the spinach into your egg bowl.
7. Scoop up 1/4 cup of the egg mixture into the muffin.
8. Sprinkle shredded cheese over the top and season it with pepper and salt
9. Bake for 15 minutes

Brie and Apple Crepes:

Makes: 4 servings

Serving size: 1 apple

Calories: 411

Preparation time: 5 minutes

Nutritional information:

Fat 37g

Protein 14g

Carbohydrates 6g

Ingredients:

1. Crepe Batter
2. 2 large eggs
3. 4 oz. cream cheese
4. Baking soda (½ tsp)
5. ¼ tsp sea salt

Topping ingredients:

1. 2 oz. chopped pecans
2. ¼ tsp cinnamon
3. 1 tbsp. unsalted butter
4. 1 small apple
5. Fresh mint leaves
6. 4 oz. brie cheese

Instructions:

1. Combine batter ingredients to blend.
2. Heat some unsalted butter on medium heat using a non-stick pan.
3. Put some crepe batter in the pan and spread it evenly. Cook for 2 minutes and turn the other side to cook as well.
4. Do this until you have 12 crepes. Place them on a plate and prepare the filling.
5. Toast the chopped pecans in a pan with some butter. Sprinkle the cinnamon and mix. Place on a plate to cool down.
6. Slice the apple and the brie cheese thinly.
7. Arrange the slices on one crepe and top it with some toasted pecans.
8. Garnish with mint lea

Steak and Eggs:

Makes: 1 serving

Serving size: 1 egg

Calories: 510

Preparation time: 10 minutes

Nutritional information:

Fat   36g

Protein 44g

Carbohydrates   3g

Ingredients:

1. 1 tbsp. butter
2. ¼ avocado
3. 3 eggs
4. Salt
5. 4 oz. sirloin
6. pepper

Instructions:

1. Melt the butter in your pan and fry three eggs. Season with pepper and salt.
2. In a different pan, cook the sirloin until desired texture. Slice into tiny strips and season it with pepper and salt.
3. Slice some avocado and serve your breakfast

Basic Oopsie Rolls

Makes: 12 servings

Serving size: 12 rolls

Calories: 45

Preparation time: 20 minutes

Nutritional information:

Fat   4g

Protein   2g

Carbohydrates   0g

Ingredients:

1. 3 large eggs
2. 1/8 tsp salt
3. 3 oz. cream cheese
4. 1/8 tsp cream tartar

Instructions:

1. Start by preheating your oven to 300°F.
2. Separate the eggs from the yolks. Place them in different mixing bowls.
3. Use an electric hand mixer to beat the egg whites until they are bubbly.
4. Add the cream of tartar and continue to beat until stiff peaks appear.
5. Add the cream cheese into the egg yolk bowl with some salt.
6. Beat until egg yolks become pale yellow.
7. Fold the egg whites and add to the cream cheese mixture.
8. Spray oil on cookie sheet and dollop the oopsie roll on it.
9. Bake for 30-40 minutes

Mini Egg Quiches

Makes: 8 servings
Serving size: 1 cup
Calories: 287
Preparation time: 10 minutes

Nutritional information:
Fat   21g
Protein   17g
Carbohydrates   4g

Ingredients:
1. 14 eggs
2. 1/3 cup pepper jack
3. 3 plum tomatoes
4. 2/3 cup mozzarella cheese
5. 2/3 cup soppressata salami
6. 1/3 cup of sweet Vidalia onion
7. 1/3 cup pickled jalapenos
8. 1 tbsp. olive oil
9. 1/3 cup heavy cream
10. 1 tsp salt
11. 1/2 tsp cayenne
12. 1 tsp pepper

Instructions:
1. Grease your muffin tin and preheat the oven to 325°F.
2. Slice and combine the ingredients in your mixing bowl.
3. Whisk the eggs until everything is mixed.
4. Add heavy cream and whisk again.
5. Mix it up
6. Put the batch on the middle rack for 25 minutes

Scrambled Eggs

Makes: 2 servings

Serving size: 1 cup

Calories: 444

Preparation time: 15 minutes

Nutritional information:

Fat   35g

Protein   25g

Carbohydrates   2g

Ingredients:

1. 6 eggs
2. 2 tbsp. sour cream
3. 2 tbsp. butter
4. 4 strips bacon
5. 2 stalks green onion
6. ½ tsp salt
7. ½ tsp onion powder
8. ½ tsp garlic powder
9. 1/4 tsp paprika
10. 1/4 tsp black pepper

Instructions:

1. Crack eggs into an ungreased pan and then add butter.
2. Use medium-high heat and stir the butter and eggs together.
3. As you stir the eggs, bake some bacon strips.
4. Alternate the stirring on and off the heat.
5. Don't stop stirring your eggs.
6. When the eggs are almost done, turn the flame off.
7. Add 2 tbsp. of crème Fraiche or sour cream.

Low Carb and Paleo Cereal

Makes: 1 serving

Serving size: 1 cup

Calories: 400

Preparation time: 5 minutes

Nutritional information:
Fat   32g
Protein   15g
Carbohydrates   7g

Ingredients:

1. ¼ cup slivered almonds
2. 1 tbsp. chia seeds
3. 2 tbsp. flaxseeds
4. 1 pinch Stevia
5. 1 tbsp. shredded coconut
6. 10 grams cocoa nibs
7. Unsweetened almond milk

Instructions:

1. Mix flax, almonds and chia seeds with the cocoa nibs and shredded coconut in a bowl.
2. Add stevia for sweetness. Pour unsweetened almond milk or flavor.

Blueberry Coconut Porridge

Makes: 2 servings

Serving size:

Calories: 405

Preparation time: 5 minutes

Nutritional information:

Fat   34g

Protein   10g

Carbohydrates   8g

Ingredients:

1. 1 cup almond milk
2. 1 pinch of salt
3. 1/4 cup coconut flour
4. 1/4 cup ground flaxseed
5. 1/4 cup coconut flour
6. 1 tsp vanilla extract
7. 1 tsp cinnamon
8. 10 drops liquid stevia

Toppings:

1. 2 tbsp. butter
2. 2 tbsp. pumpkin seeds
3. 60 grams blueberries
4. 1 oz. shaved coconut

Instructions:

1. Heat up some almond milk on a low flame.
2. Mix coconut flour, flaxseed, salt and cinnamon in the milk.
3. Heat until it bubbles slightly. Add vanilla extract and stevia.
4. When it reaches your desired thickness, turn off the flame.
5. Add your toppings.

Fat-Burning Vanilla Smoothie

Makes: 1 serving

Serving size: 10 oz.

Calories: 650

Preparation time: 2 minutes

Nutritional information:

Fat   64g

Protein   12g

Carbohydrates 4g

Ingredients:

1. 1/4 cup water
2. 2 large egg yolks
3. 4 ice cubes
4. 1/2 cup mascarpone cheese
5. 1 tbsp. coconut oil
6. 1 tbsp. powdered erythritol
7. 1/2 tsp pure vanilla extract
8. whipped cream

Instructions:

1. Use a blender and mix the mascarpone, egg yolks, water, creamed coconut milk, MCT, and other ingredients. Pulse until the mix is smooth.

2. Top it with whipped cream.

Salad recipes

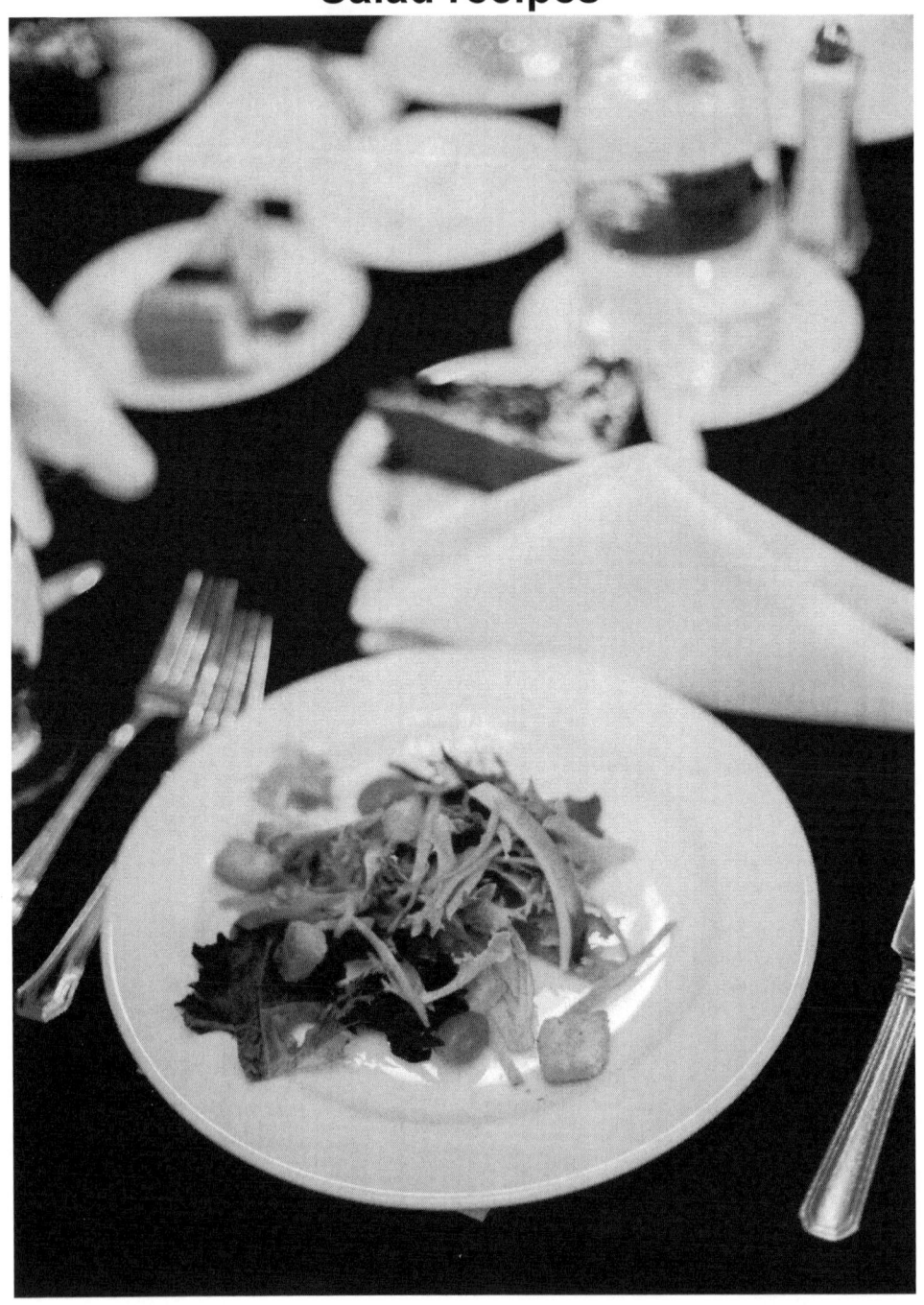

Strawberry Cheesecake Salad:

Makes: 4 servings

Serving size: 1 salad

Calories: 72

Preparation time: 15 minutes

Nutritional information:

Fat   0.2 g

Protein   1.8 g

Carbohydrates 14.2g

Ingredients:

1. 1/2 cup heavy cream
2. 8oz cream cheese
3. 10g freeze dried strawberries
4. 2 tbsp. sugar-free sweetening syrup
5. 1/4 cup almond flour
6. 8 oz. fresh strawberries

Instructions:

1. Put half cream and cream cheese into an automatic mixer bowl and mix on the slow setting.
2. Add you sweetening syrup and freeze-dried strawberry powder and mix.
3. Add the almond flour and fresh strawberries, and stir by hand.
4. Serve in a dish and enjoy.

Curried Cabbage Coconut Salad

Makes: 2 servings

Serving size: 1 salad

Calories: 309

Preparation time: 2 minutes

Nutritional information:

Fat   29g

Protein 5g

Carbohydrates   35g

Fiber   21g

Ingredients:

1. 1 Lemon Juice
2. 1/2 head White cabbage
3. 1/3 cup Dried coconut unsweetened
4. 1/4 cup Tamari sauce
5. 1/4 cup coconut oil
6. 1/2 teaspoon ginger, dried
7. 3 teaspoons sesame seeds
8. 1/2 teaspoon cumin
9. 1/2 teaspoon curry powder

Instructions:

1. Add all the ingredients in a mixing bowl and mix.
2. Chill for one hour
3. Enjoy your salad

Coconut & Turmeric Chia Pudding

Makes: 1 serving

Serving size: 1 salad

Calories: 833

Preparation time: 5 minutes

Nutritional information:

Fat   78g

Proteins   12g

Carbohydrates   35g

Fiber   21g

Ingredients:

1. 2 tbsp. chia seeds
2. 1/2 tin coconut milk
3. 1/4 tbsp. ground cardamom
4. 1 inch fresh turmeric
5. 1/2 cup unsweetened dried coconut.

Instructions:

1. Start by mixing the spices, chia seeds, and desiccated coconut.
2. Add your coconut milk and blend.
3. Store in a container in the fridge until morning.

Halloumi Stuffed Peppers

Makes: 1 serving

Serving size: 1 salad

Calories: 198

Preparation time: 30 minutes

Nutritional information:

Fat   15g

Protein   10g

Carbohydrates 6g

Fiber   2g

Ingredients:

1. 2 tbsp. Olive oil
2. 3 Red Peppers
3. 12 Mint leaves torn
4. 3 Garlic Cloves chopped
5. 1 tablespoon Thyme
6. 250 grams Halloumi Cheese
7. One Lemon - Grated and Rind

Instructions:

1. Start by preheating your oven 400F degrees.
2. Slice the peppers in half and remove the seeds and core.
3. Rub oil on the pepper skin and arrange them on a greased baking tray.
4. Sprinkle some garlic in the peppers and add cheese, mint leaves, lemon rind, thyme and garlic.
5. Pour the lemon juice and oil over the mix.
6. Roast for about 30 minutes.

Feta Lemon Coleslaw

Makes: 2 servings

Serving size: I salad

Calories: 165

Preparation time: 5 minutes

Nutritional information:

Fat   14g

Protein 4g

Carbohydrates   7g

Fiber   2g

Ingredients:

1. ½ cup Lemon juice
2. 1/2 White cabbage
3. 3 tablespoons Olive oil
4. 2 Spring onions
5. 1/2 cup Feta cheese
6. 1/2 teaspoon Black pepper
7. 1/2 teaspoon Salt

Instructions:

1. Put the cabbage and onion in the bowl.
2. Blend your lemon, Feta cheese, and olive oil in the bowl. Add salt and pepper.
3. Add cabbage.

Greek Goddess Kale Salad

Makes: 12 servings

Serving size: 1 salad

Calories: 99

Preparation time: 15 minutes

Nutritional information:

Fat   7.2g

Protein   2.5g

Carbohydrates 6.5g

Ingredients:

1. 1/4 cup sliced red onion
2. 6 cups fresh kale
3. 1 cup sliced cucumber
4. 1/4 cup red onion
5. 1/2 cup cherry tomatoes
6. 1/4 cup kalamata olives
7. 1/4 cup pine nuts

Greek Goddess Dressing:

1. 3 cloves of garlic
2. 1 lemon juice
3. 8 ounces Organic sour cream
4. 21g fresh basil
5. .50 ounce fresh chives
6. 1 ounce fresh parsley
7. Pepper and salt

Instructions:

1. Clean the kale and slice. Place in a salad bowl.
2. Place the salad ingredients, except the pine nuts on the kale.
3. Toast your pine nuts using a dry skillet over medium-high heat. Sprinkle it over the salad.
4. Make the dressing in the blender
5. The must be poured into the blender first.
6. Add other ingredients
7. Blend and taste it to know if you want extra salt and pepper.

Summer Confetti Salad

Makes: 1 serving

Serving size: 1 salad

Calories: 109

Preparation time: 5 minutes

Nutritional information:

Fat   9g

Protein   2g

Carbohydrates   7g

Ingredients:

1. 1/4 cup chopped scallions
2. 3 cups chopped cauliflower
3. 1/2 cup chopped red bell pepper
4. 1/3 cup chopped yellow bell pepper
5. 1 cup finely chopped red cabbage
6. 1/2 cup finely chopped celery
7. 1/4 cup fresh basil

Dressing Ingredients:

1. 2 tsp fresh lime juice
2. 1/4 cup avocado oil
3. 2 Tbsp. of apple cider vinegar
4. 1/2 tsp kosher salt
5. 1 ½ Tbsp. fresh ginger
6. 2 Tbsp. granulated sweetener

Instructions:

1. Mix the chopped veggies in a salad bowl.
2. Combine dressing ingredients in your magic bullet and blend for 30 seconds.
3. Mix the dressing with the salad

Amish Broccoli Cauliflower Salad

Makes: 7 servings

Serving size: 1 cup

Calories: 324

Preparation Time: 20 minutes

Nutritional information:

Fat   32g

Protein   7g

Carbohydrates   5g

Fiber   2g

Ingredients:

1. 8 oz. broccoli florets
2. 8 oz. cauliflower florets
3. 2 oz. red bell pepper
4. 4 oz. cheddar cheese
5. 1/3 pound cooked bacon
6. 2 tbsp. purple onion

Dressing:

1. 3/4 cup sour cream
2. 3/4 cup mayonnaise
3. 1 tbsp. lemon juice
4. 2 tbsp. stevia

Instructions:

1. Slice bacon and cook in a frying pan until crisp.
2. Wash and chop your vegetables and put them in a large bowl.
3. Mix the dressing ingredients in a medium bowl.
4. Toss the salad ingredients and stir into the dressing

Cucumber Salad (Thai)

Makes: 4 servings

Serving size: I salad

Calories: 75

Preparation Time: 15 minutes

Nutritional information:

Fat   5g

Protein 6g

Carbohydrates 5g

Fiber   2g

Ingredients:

1. 2-3 scallions
2. 16 ounces cucumber, peeled
3. 1/4 cup chopped cilantro

Dressing:

1. 1 tbsp. water
2. 1/4 cup white vinegar
3. 1 tbsp. toasted sesame oil
4. 1/4 cup Icing Sugar
5. 1 tbsp. sesame seeds
6. 1 tbsp. Fish Sauce
7. 1/2 teaspoon salt
8. Thai red chilies
9. Carrots, grated
10. Purple cabbage

Instructions:

1. Peel the cucumber and slice into 1/2 rounds.
2. Slice the scallion, and chop the cilantro.
3. Slice all other toppings.
4. Cover and refrigerate.

For the Dressing:

1. Add all dressing ingredients in a bowl. Stir to dissolve yo

Grilled Chicken Breast Salad

Makes: 1 serving

Serving size:1salad

Calories: 302

Preparation Time: 10 minutes

Nutritionalinformation:

Fat21

Protein 21g

Carbohydrates 8g

Fiber 3g

Ingredients:
1. 1-ounce fennel bulb
2. 70g arugula
3. 1-ounce cherry
4. 1-ounce red bell
5. 1-ounce cucumber sliced
6. 3 ounces Garlic
7. Herb Grilled Chicken
8. 1 serving Garlic/Herb Vinaigrette

Instructions:
1. Slice all the ingredients.
2. Throw in the greens with your salad dressing.
3. Place protein first, and fill-in with other ingredients.

Soup recipes

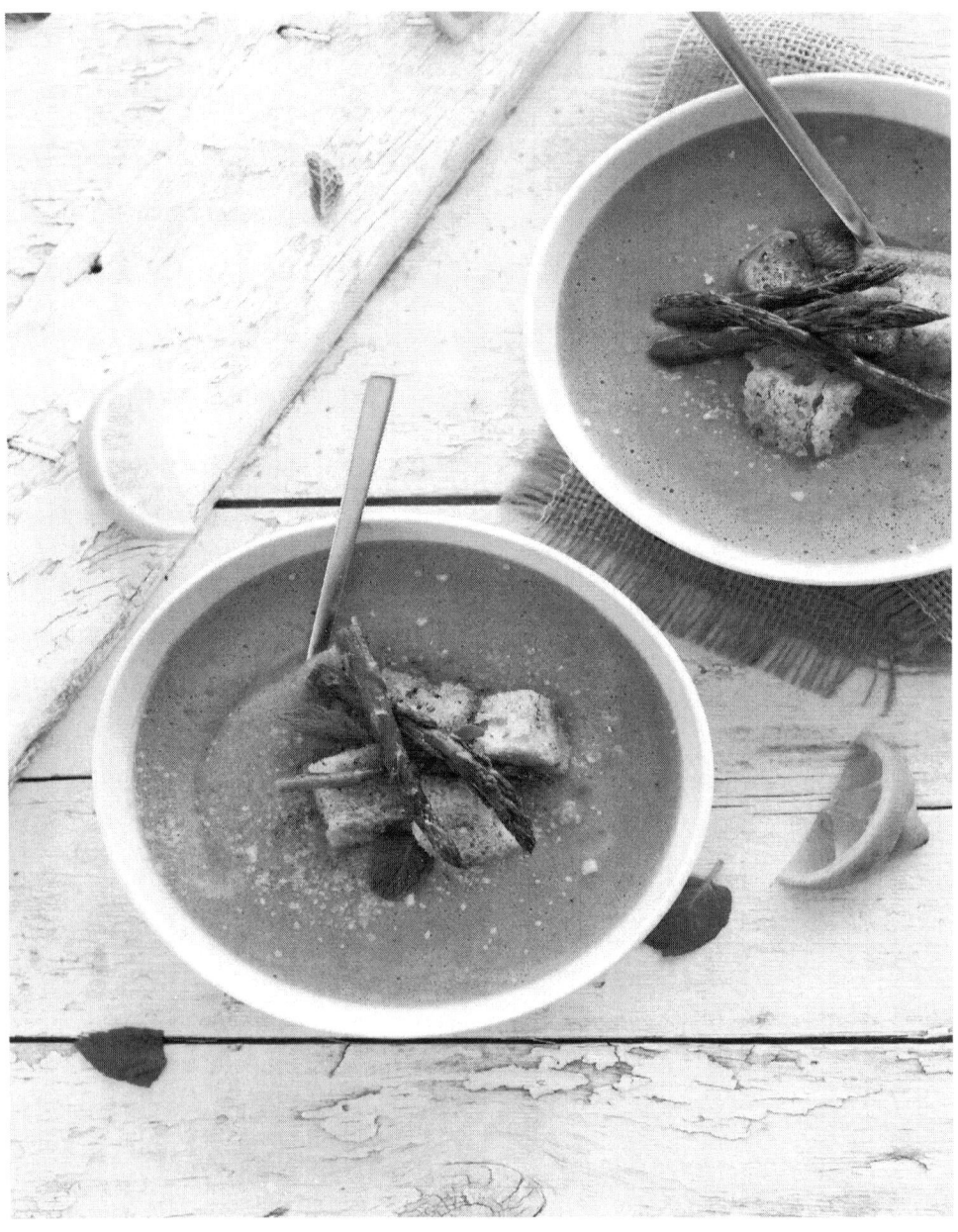

Ham and Green Bean Soup:

Makes: 12 servings

Serving size: 1 cup

Calories: 158 kcal

Nutritional information:

Fat 7g

Protein 11g

Carbohydrates 12g

Ingredients:

1. quart chicken broth
1. 1-quart ham broth
2. 2 cups water
3. 2 cloves garlic (chopped
4. 2 tablespoons bacon dripping
5. 1 pound green beans
6. 3 ounces onion
7. 1 pound red potatoes
8. Salt and pepper
10. 1 pound ham
11. 1/2 tbsp. garlic powder
12. 1/2 tbsp. liquid smoke flavoring

Instructions:

1. Slice the garlic and onion and heat the bacon medium heat.
2. Sauté the garlic and onions in the oil until they become translucent.
3. Pour the chicken and ham broths into a pot with water.
4. Add green beans and allow to cook. Add the salt, potatoes, liquid smoke flavoring as well as the garlic powder.
5. Add the ham and continue to heat.
6. Adjust your seasoning and serve.

Cauliflower and ham soup

Makes: 10 servings

Serving size: 1 cup

Calories: 125

Preparation time: 30 minutes

Nutritional information:

Fat   7g

Protein   13g

Carbohydrates   5g

Ingredients:

1. 2 cups water
2. 6 cups cauliflower florets
3. 6 cups chicken broth
4. 1/2 tsp onion powder
5. 1/2 tsp garlic powder
6. 3 cups chopped ham
7. 1 Tbsp. thyme leaves
8. 2 Tbsp. butter
9. 2 Tbsp. apple cider vinegar

Instructions:

1. Mix the stock, cauliflower, water, onion and garlic powder in a large pot.
2. Boil for 20-30 minutes.
3. Blend in pot using an immersion blender until smooth.
4. Add the thyme leaves and ham and simmer 10 minutes.
5. Put the apple cider vinegar and butter.
6. Put it down and season with pepper and salt.

Moqueca De Camaroes

Makes: 6 servings

Serving size: 1 cup

Calories: 294

Preparation time: 30 minutes

Nutritional information: Fat 19g

Protein 24g

Carbohydrates 5g

Ingredients:

1. 1/4 cup olive oil
2. 1 1/2 lbs. raw shrimp
3. 1/4 cup onion, diced
4. 1/4 cup red pepper, roasted
5. 1 clove garlic, minced
6. 1 cup coconut milk
7. 1/4 cup fresh cilantro
8. 14 oz. diced tomatoes
9. 2 Tbsp. Sriracha hot sauce
10. 2 Tbsp. lime juice
11. Pepper and salt

Instructions:

1. In str olive oil in a saucepan and sauté the onions until translucent.
2. Add the peppers, garlic, and cook.
3. Add the shrimp, tomatoes, and cilantro and simmer gently.
4. Pour the sriracha sauce and coconut milk and cook until heated.
5. Pour the lime juice and salt and pepper.

Roasted Broccoli & Cheddar Soup

Makes: 4 servings

Serving size: 1 cup

Calories: 223

Preparation time: 10 minutes

Nutritional information:

Fat   11.3g

Protein   16.8g

Carbohydrates   14.1g

Fiber 3.2g

Ingredients:

1. 1 tbsp. oil
2. 1 large bunch broccoli
3. salt and pepper
4. 1 medium onion
5. 1 teaspoon thyme
6. 2 cloves garlic
7. 3 cups chicken broth
8. 1 ½ cups aged cheddar
9. 1 tbsp. grainy mustard
10. 1 cup cream
11. Salt and pepper

Instructions:

1. Throw in the broccoli florets with salt and pepper in oil and bake until lightly golden brown.
2. Heat the oil and add the onion and sauté until it is tender.
3. Add the thyme, garlic, and sauté until fragrant.
4. Add the broccoli and broth, boil, reduce heat and then simmer. Cover for about 20 minutes.
5. Add cheese, milk, and mustard.
6. Mash the soup using a hand blender.

Avgolemono soup

Makes: 8 servings

Serving size: 1.5 cups Calories: 289

Preparation time: 20 minutes

Nutritional information:

Fat 15g

Protein 33g,

Carbohydrates   4g

Ingredients:

1. 3 eggs
2. 4 cups cooked chicken
3. 10 cups chicken stock
4. 1/4 cup fresh parsley
5. 1/3 cup lemon juice
6. 2 cups spaghetti squash, cooked
7. Pepper and salt

Instructions:

1. Place the broth in a saucepan and boil it.
2. Use a medium bowl to whisk the lemon juice and eggs together until foamy.
3. Whisk 2 cups of stock into the mixture. It should be hot. Add it to the pot.
4. Add the spaghetti squash.
5. Season with pepper and salt.

Jalapeno popper soup

Makes: 4 servings

Serving size: 1 cup

Calories: 425

Preparation time: 20 minutes

Nutritional information:

Fat   38g

Protein   17g

Carbohydrates   2.5g

Ingredients:

1. 4 oz. cream cheese
2. 4 slices raw bacon
3. 2 tbsp. salsa verde
4. 1/2 cup heavy cream
5. 1/2 tsp garlic powder
6. 2 cups chicken broth
7. 4 large jalapeno peppers
8. 3/4 cup sliced sharp cheddar cheese
9. 1/4 tsp xanthan gum
10. 3/4 cup sliced Monterey jack cheese

Instructions:

1. Start by cooking the bacon until crisp.
2. Add water, heavy cream, and cream cheese.
3. Boil gently, stirring, until your cream cheese melts completely.
4. Add the salsa verde, garlic powder, and shredded cheeses.
5. Wash the jalapenos and grill them until charred.
6. Remove the seeds and skins and chop finely.
7. Pour into the soup. Cook for 5 minutes.

Mulligatawny Soup

Makes: 10 servings

Serving size: 1 cup

Calories: 214

Preparation time: 30 min

Nutritional information

Fat 4g

Protein 36g

Carbohydrate 4g

Ingredients:

1 ½ Tbsp. curry powder

1. 10 cups chicken broth
2. 2 Tbsp. Swerve sweetener
3. 5 cups chopped chicken
4. 3 cups celery root
5. 1/4 cup juice or apple cider
6. 1/2 cup sour cream
7. Pepper and salt
8. 1/4 cup fresh parsley

Instructions

1. Mix the curry powder, broth, chicken, apple cider vinegar and celery root rice in a large pot.
2. Boil for 30 minutes.
3. Pour the sour cream, sweetener, and fresh parsley.
4. Season with pepper and salt

Pumpkin Chipotle Soup

Makes: 6 servings

Serving size: one cup

Calories: 138

Preparation time:

Nutritional information:

Fat   12g

Protein   9g

Carbohydrates   6g

Ingredients:

1. 1/2 cup chopped onions
2. 2 Tbsp. olive oil
3. 1 clove garlic
4. 1 Tbsp. chipotles
5. 1 tsp ground cumin
6. 1 tsp ground coriander
7. 2 cups pumpkin puree
8. 1/8 tsp ground allspice
9. 32 oz. chicken broth
10. 2 tbsp. granulated sugar
11. 2 tsp red wine vinegar
12. 1/2 cup heavy cream
13. Pepper and salt

Instructions:

1. Heat your olive oil and sauté garlic and onions for 3 minutes until they're translucent.
2. Add the cumin, chipotles, coriander, allspice, as well as a sugar substitute to the saucepan and cook for 2 minutes.
3. Add your chicken broth and pumpkin puree to the pot and let it simmer for 5 minutes.
4. Use an immersion blender to blend the soup until smooth
5. Add red wine vinegar and heavy cream and simmer for five minute

Cream of tomato soup

Makes: I serving

Serving size: 1cup

Calories: 187

Preparation time: 5min

Fat   15.9g

Protein   3.5 g

Carbohydrates   11.8 g

Fiber   4.1 g

Ingredients:

1. 1 teaspoon sea salt
2. 4 Roma tomatoes
3. ½ cup sun-dried tomatoes
4. ¼ cup fresh basil
5. ½ cup macadamia nuts, raw
6. ½ teaspoon white pepper
7. 1 clove garlic
8. ¼ teaspoon black pepper
9. 4 cups hot water

Instructions:

1. Put all ingredients in a high-powered blender. Blend for 5 minutes on high until heated.
2. Serve and enjoy.
10. ½ teaspoon white pepper
11. 1 clove garlic
12. ¼ teaspoon black pepper
13. 4 cups hot water

Instructions:

3. Put all ingredients in a high-powered blender. Blend for 5 minutes on high until heated.
4. Serve and enjoy.

Greens Cream Soup

Makes: 4 servings

Serving size: 1 cup

Calories: 95

Preparation time: 5 minutes

Nutritional information:

Fat   7.6g

Protein 2.1 g

Carbohydrates   6.7 g

Fiber   4.2 g

Ingredients:

1. 1 avocado
2. 2 cups spinach leaves
3. 1/2 cup English cucumber
4. 1 clove garlic
5. 1 green onion
6. ½ cup pepper, red bell
7. 1/4 cup vegetable broth
8. 1 tbsp. lemon juice
9. 1 tbsp. soy seasoning
10. Freshly ground pepper
11. Pinch chili powder

Instructions:

1. Blend all ingredients until smooth.
2. Serve and enjoy

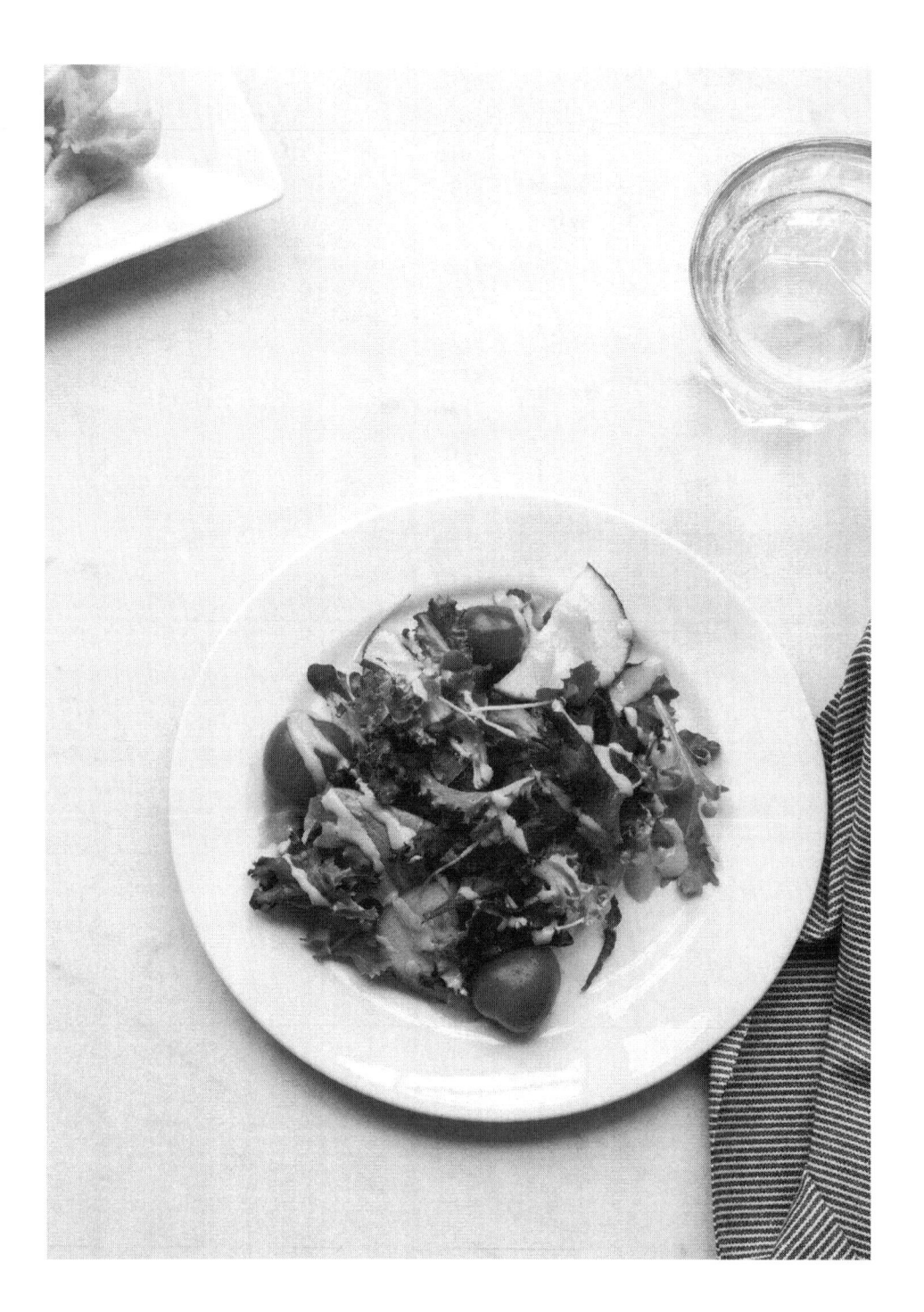

Lunch recipes

Salami rollups

Makes: 1 serving

Serving size: 1 cup

Calories: 564

Preparation time: 1 minute

Nutritional information:

Fat 51g

Protein   22.5g

Carbohydrates 2.9g

Ingredients:

1. 1 handful of rocket leaves
2. 8 salami slices (40g)
3. 80g cream cheese
4. 2 slices of Protein Bread (optional)
5. 20g Kerrygold softer butter

Instructions:

1. Toast bread slices and butter them (optional).
2. Spread the salami slices and place some cheese on them.
3. Top with rocket leaves and then roll up.
4. Serve and enjoy.

Protein roll

Makes: 1 serving

Serving size: 1 roll

Calories: 410

Preparation time: 6 minutes

Nutritional information:

Fat	36g
Protein	17g
Carbohydrates	2.9g

Ingredients:

1. ½ tbsp. hummus
2. 3 slices Halloumi cheese
3. 5 green olives
4. 2 knobs Kerrygold softer butter
5. 2 Little Gem leaves
6. 1 Low Carb Protein Bread Roll

Instructions:

1. Shallow fry the cheese until the water evaporates as well as the Halloumi.
2. Cut the bread roll horizontally and toast.
3. Put the Halloumi on the Little Gem lettuce.
4. Add hummus and spoon olives to your serving plate.

Avocado burrata and cheese chips

Makes: 1 serving

Serving size: 1

Calories: 953

Preparation time: 2 minutes

Nutritional information:

Fat   67.5g

Protein   55.3g

Carbohydrates   1.9g

Ingredients:

1. 80g avocado
2. 1 (200g) burrata
3. 100g low carb cheese

Instructions:

1. Slice the cheese and avocado.
2. Remove the burrata from its tub and place alongside avocado slices and cheese chips.

Cheese and ham toasted sandwich

Makes: 1 serving

Serving size: 1

Calories: 774

Preparation time: 5 minutes

Nutritional information:

Fat   65g

Protein   43g

Carbohydrates   3g

Ingredients:

1. 4 slices Low Carb Protein Bread
2. 4 slices mature Cheddar
3. 2 knobs Kerrygold softer butter
4. 1 squirt low carb mayonnaise
5. Some strands of cucumber

Instructions:

1. Toast the bread slices and then butter them.
2. Add cheese and prosciutto
3. Serve with mayonnaise or some cucumber strands.

Avocado salad, prawns, and toasted bread

Makes: 1 serving

Serving size: 1

Calories: 336

Preparation time: 5 minutes

Nutritional information:

Fat   25g

Protein   22.5g

Carbohydrates   3g

Ingredients:

1. 40g avocado
2. 100g cooked and skinned prawns
3. 20g low carb mayonnaise
4. 1 tsp lemon juice
5. A drop of Worcestershire sauce
6. 1 squirt tomato concentrate
7. a pinch of Himalayan pink salt
8. 1 pinch paprika
9. 2 knobs Kerrygold softer butter
10. 2 slices Low Carb Protein Bread

Instructions:

1. Mix diced avocado, prawns, lemon juice, mayonnaise, salt, Worcestershire sauce and paprika in a medium bowl.
2. Mix with a fork.
3. Pour some cold water.
4. Taste and add salt/paprika.
4. Pour on Little Gem Lettuce.

Bacon whiskey caramelized onions

Makes: 1 serving

Serving size: 1

Calories: 262.1

Preparation time: 20 minutes

Nutritional information:

Fat   8.2

Protein   20.2g

Carbohydrates   10g

Ingredients:

1. 1 tbsp. Bacon grease
2. 1 onion
3. Water
4. 1 tbsp. Whiskey

Instructions:

1. Heat the bacon with a pan on medium heat.
2. Cut the onions into long slices.
3. Put the onion slices on the pan and cook.
4. Mix and add some whiskey when it sticks.
5. Turn with 1 tbsp. water until onions turn brown.

Tamari Marinated Steak Salad

Makes: 2 servings

Serving size: 2

Calories: 500

Preparation time: 20 minutes

Nutritional Information:

Fat   37 g

Protein   33 g

Carbohydrates   4 g

Fiber   2 g

Ingredients:

1. 4 radishes, sliced
2. 2 large handfuls salad greens
3. 1 tbsp. olive oil
4. ½ red bell pepper, sliced
5. 6-8 cherry tomatoes, chopped
6. ½ tbsp. fresh lemon juice
7. Salt
8. Olive or avocado oil
9. ½ lb. steak
10. ¼ cup tamari soy sauce

Instructions:

1. Marinade your steak in tamari soy sauce.
2. Start preparing the salad by tossing in tomatoes, bell pepper, radishes, as well as salad greens. Add lemon juice, olive oil, and salt.
3. Divide the salad and place into 2 plates.
4. Put the avocado oil in a frying pan and cook your marinated steak.
5. Remove the steak and place it on a plate for a minute. Slice the steak into thin slices, and put half on top each salad.

Chicken Bites

Makes: 4 servings

Serving size: 1

Calories: 230

Preparation time: 15 minutes

Nutritional information:

Fat 13 g

Protein 22 g

Carbohydrates 5 g

Fiber 1 g

Ingredients:

1. Preheat your oven to 400F and line the baking tray with an aluminum foil.
2. Put the garlic powder in a bowl and place each chicken bite in the garlic powder.
3. Pack each bacon piece around the garlic chicken bite. Put the bacon wrapped bites on your baking tray. Ensure that you space them out to prevent them from touching.
4. Bake for about 25-30 minutes until your bacon becomes crispy. Remember to turn the pieces after about 15 minutes.

Mustard Sardines Salad

Makes: 1 serving

Serving size: 1

Calories: 260

Preparation time: 5 minutes

Nutritional information:

Fat   20g

Protein   25g

Carbohydrates   0g

Ingredients:

1. 1 tbsp. lemon juice
2. 1 can sardine in olive oil
3. ¼ cucumber
4. ½ Tablespoon mustard
5. Pepper and salt.

Instructions:

1. Drain the olive oil from your sardines.
2. Puree the sardines.
3. Mix the diced cucumbers, sardines, lemon juice, salt, mustard, and pepper.

Mini Zucchini Avocado Burgers

Makes: 2 servings

Serving size : 2

Calories: 370

Preparation time: 15 minutes

Nutritional information:

Fat   30 g

Protein   23 g

Carbohydrates   9 g

Fiber   6 g

Ingredients:

1. ½ lb. ground beef
2. 1 large zucchini, sliced into ½-inch thick slices. It would make 14-16 slices.
3. ¼ avocado, chopped into small slices.
4. 2 Tablespoons avocado or olive oil to grease the baking tray.
5. 1 tbsp. Paleo mayo
6. 2 teaspoons salt
7. 1 Tablespoon mustard

Instructions:

1. Preheat oven to 400F.
2. Grease a baking tray with olive or avocado oil and sprinkle 1 teaspoon of salt across it.
3. Put the zucchini slices on your baking tray.
4. Create small balls from your ground beef and make them into patties. You can make 7 or 8 patties. Place on your baking tray.
5. Put the baking tray in the oven and let it bake for about 15 minutes. If you do not want to bake them, you can opt to grill the beef patties and zucchini or pan-fry them the beef in avocado or olive oil.
6. In the meantime, slice your avocado into tiny thin slices.
7. Place the mini burgers in one place using your zucchini slices as buns. Next, add one slice of avocado on each burger and cover it with condiments such   as mustard and Paleo mayo.

Dessert recipes

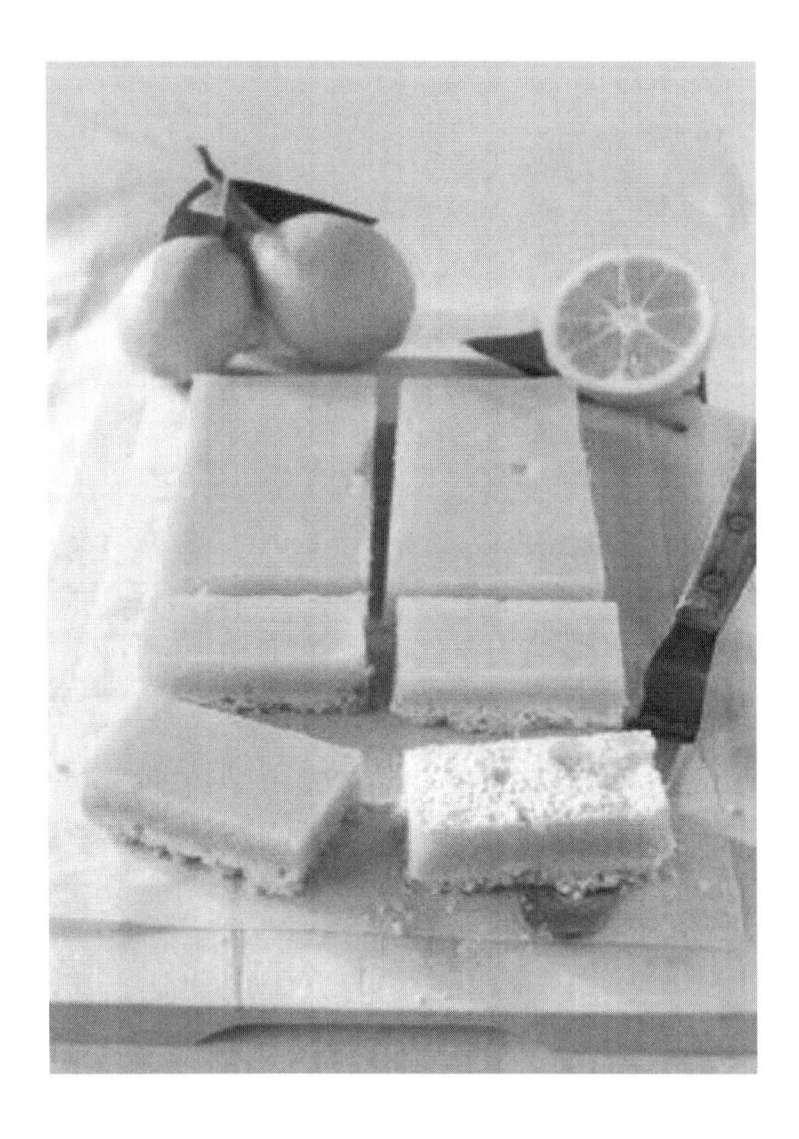

Coconut Oil Candies

Makes: 1 serving

Serving size: I cup

Calories: 73

Preparation time: 20 minutes

Nutritional information:

Fat 7 g

Protein 1g

Carbohydrates 0.9g

Ingredients:

1. 1 cup virgin coconut oil
2. 1/2 tsp Celtic Sea Salt
3. 1 tsp vanilla extract
4. 1-2 Tbsp. sweetener
5. 2-4 Tbsp. unsweetened cocoa powder
6. 2 Tbsp. nut butter

Instructions:

1. Mix ingredients in a bowl until the mixture is smooth.
2. Place by the tablespoon on parchment paper

Chocolate Ice Cream

Makes: 2 servings

Serving size: 1 cup

Calories: 318

Preparation time: 5 minutes

Nutritional information:

Fat   28.6g

Protein   3g

Carbohydrates   9.1g

Ingredients:

1. 1-teaspoon chocolate stevia
2. 1 can coconut milk
3. Pinch of salt
4. 2 tablespoons unsweetened cocoa powder
5. cacao nibs

Instructions:

1. Mix all ingredients in the blender.
1. Pour mixture into the ice cream machine. Follow the manufacturer's instructions.

Instant Avocado Vanilla Pudding

Makes: 1 serving

Serving size: 1 cup

Calories: 284

Preparation time: 5 minutes

Nutritional information:

Fat   23g

Protein   7g

Carbohydrates   24g

Fiber   18g

Ingredients:

1. 80 drops liquid stevia
2. 1 can organic coconut milk
3. 2 teaspoons vanilla extract
4. 1 tablespoon lime juice
5. 2 ripe avocados

Instructions:

1. Add ingredients to your blender.
2. Blend until it is smooth and velvety.

Sugar-free Lemon Curd

Makes: 1 serving

Serving size: 1 cup

Calories: 98

Preparation time: 5

Nutritional information

Fat 10g

Protein 1g

Carbohydrates 1g

Ingredients:

1. 1/2 cup lemon juice
2. 1/2 cup butter
3. 1/2 cup xylitol sweetener
4. 6 egg yolks
5. 1/4 cup lemon zest

Instructions:

1. Melt butter in a saucepan using low heat.
2. Whisk in lemon juice, sweetener, and lemon zest until it dissolves.
3. Whisk in egg yolks and take it back to the stove.
4. Whisk repeatedly until the curd thickens.
5. Remove from stove and strain in a small bowl

Lemon cloud pie

Makes: 8 servings

Serving size: 1/8 pie

Calories: 427

Preparation time: 20 minutes

Nutritional information:

Fat   46g

Protein   4g

Carbohydrates   2.5g

Ingredients:

1. 3/4 cup almond flour
2. 6 Tbsp. butter
3. 3/4 cup erythritol
4. 3/4 cup dried coconut
5. A pinch of salt

Filling:

1. ¼ cup lemon zest
2. ½ cup butter
3. ½ cup erythritol
4. ½ cup lemon juice
5. 6 egg yolks
6. 1/4 tsp xanthan gum
7. 1 1/2 cups heavy whipping cream

Instructions:

1. Mix the erythritol, butter, coconut, salt and almond flour in a bowl and mix.
2. Put the dough in a pie plate.
3. Bake the piecrust at 350 degrees for 15 minutes.
4. Melt butter in a saucepan on low heat.
5. Take it down and whisk in lemon juice, sweetener, and lemon zest.
6. Add the egg yolks and place it on low heat.
7. Whisk and remove from the heat. Strain into a bowl. Chill.
8. Whip the xanthan gum, heavy whipping cream, sweetener together until stiff.
9. Fold some whipped cream mix into the cold lemon curd until blended.
10. Add the lighter lemon curd mixture and gently fold together.
11. Scoop the filling onto the cooled piecrust and garnish with lemon zest and whipped cream.

Fresh Fruit Tart

Makes: 12 servings

Serving size: 1cup

Calories: 272

Preparation time: 20   minutes

Nutritional information:

Fat   25g

Protein   5g

Carbohydrates   10g

Ingredients:

1. 3 ripe kiwi fruit
2. 1 Fresh Fruit Garnish
3. 6 large blackberries
4. 6 ounces fresh blueberries
5. 18 raspberries

Instructions:

1. Make your Coconut Milk Pastry Cream 5 days before the Fresh Fruit Tarts.
2. Make your Almond-Coconut Tart Crust.
3. Remove your cold pastry cream from the fridge and stir.
4. Line the tart shells on a baking sheet.
5. Wash and dry your fruit.
6. Put some pastry cream in the tart shell and smoothen it.
7. Set the blackberry right in the middle and put three raspberries around it.
8. Place the blueberries in the vacant space

No-Bake Rhubarb Crisp

Makes: 4 servings

Serving size: 1 cup

Calories: 273

Preparation time: 8 minutes

Nutritional information:

Fat   26g

Protein   7g

Carbohydrates   5g

Ingredients:

1. ¼ cup unsweetened almond milk
2. ⅔ cup diced rhubarb
3. ⅛ teaspoon sea salt
4. 1 cream cheese.
5. ⅓ cup Swerve confectioners
6. 1 teaspoon vanilla extract
7. ½ cup crushed almonds

Instructions:

1. Put the rhubarb in your bowl and microwave for about 2 minutes.
2. Add cashew milk, cream cheese, salt, natural sweetener, and extract and stir.
3. Add to 4 ramekins and smoothen the top.

Strawberry Cream Pie

Makes: 10 servings

Serving size: 1 pie

Calories: 348

Preparation time: 20 minutes

Nutritional information:

Fat   30g

Protein 13g

Carbohydrates   10g

Ingredients:

1. 1 tablespoon lemon juice
2. 1 cup Fage Yogurt
3. Swerve Confectioners
4. 1/2 teaspoon vanilla extract
5. 1.2 ounce dried strawberries
6. 1/4 teaspoon strawberry extract
7. 1 cup heavy cream
8. 1 pinch salt

Instructions:

1. Prepare the pie crust.
2. Measure all ingredients, except whipped cream, and mix with hand mixer.
3. Whip your heavy cream until stiff.
4. Add some whipped cream into your strawberry yogurt mixture.
5. Mix with mixer until combined.
6. Add some cream into the cream mixture and fold with a rubber spatula.
7. Pour the strawberry cream filling on the pie crust.
8. Smoothen the edges and the top.

Cheesecake Salad

Makes: 23 servings Serving size: 1 cup Calories: 134 calories Preparation time: 10 minutes Nutritional information: Fat 11g

Protein 8g

Carbohydrates 2g

Ingredients:

1. 1/4 teaspoon stevia
2. 16 ounces cream cheese
3. 1 cup heavy whipped cream
4. 1/2 teaspoon of monk fruit concentrated powder
5. 16 ounces strawberries
6. 14 ounces blueberries
7. 12 ounces blackberries
8. 6 ounces raspberries

Instructions:

1. Beat the cream cheese using an electric mixer.

2. Add the stevia, monk fruit, and heavy whipped cream.

3. Beat it with electric mixer until creamy and thick.

Cherry Chocolate Cheesecake

Makes: 8 servings

Serving size: 1 cup

Calories: 185

Preparation time: 45minutes

Nutritional information:

Fat   16.8g

Protein   2.7g

Carbohydrates   10.4g

Ingredients:

1. 1 cup heavy cream
2. 4 ounces cream cheese
3. 1 cup sour cream
4. 1/4 cup Swerve
5. 1/8 teaspoon stevia
6. 1/8 teaspoon of monk fruit powder
7. 1/2 teaspoon lemon extract
8. 1 teaspoon cherry extract
9. 3 tablespoons cocoa 10. 1/4 teaspoon vanilla extract

Instructions:

1. Beat the cream cheese and sweeteners.
2. Add the sour cream, heavy cream, and cocoa until smooth.
3. Add the extracts.
4. Cover it and place in the fridge for 2-3 hours.
5. Beat until creamy.
6. Place in an ice cream maker. Process until satisfied.

Meat recipes

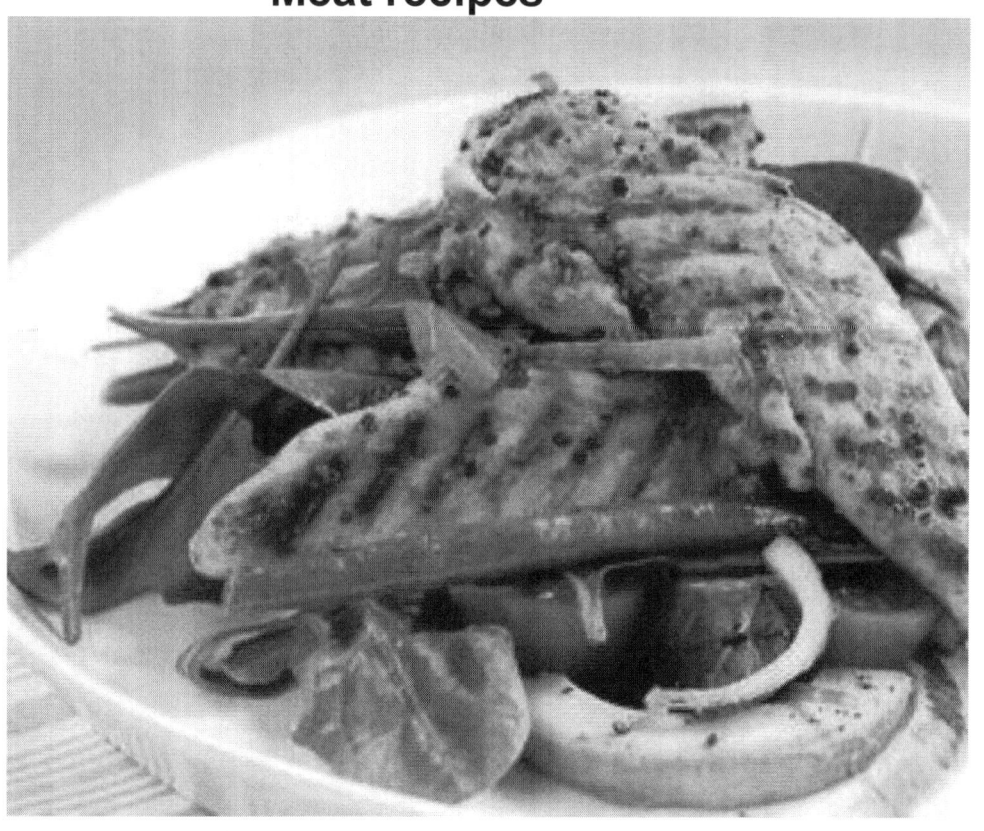

Corned beef hash

Makes: 4 servings

Serving size: 6 oz.

Calories: 506

Preparation time: 30 minutes

Nutritional information:

Fat   43.2g

Protein   22g

Carbohydrates   16.08g

Ingredients:

1. 2 cloves garlic
2. 2 cups chopped corned beef
3. 1/2 cup beef broth
4. 1 small onion
5. Pepper and salt
6. 1 lb. radishes

Instructions:

1. Heat up 1 Tbsp. oil over medium heat.
2. Pour the onions and sauté them for 3-4 minutes.
3. Put the radishes next and sauté for about 5 minutes.
4. Put the garlic and sauté for 1 minute.
5. Pour in the beef broth and cook.
6. Add the corned beef.
7. Season with salt and stir to combine

Low Carb Beef Burritos

Makes: 6 servings

Serving size: 6.5 crepes

Calories: 235

Preparation time: 10 minutes

Nutritional information:

Fat   19.4g

Protein   10.2g

Carbohydrate   5.5g

Ingredients:

1. Mince Beef 500 g
2. 1 red onion
3. 1 tbsp. ground cumin
4. 2 cloves garlic crushed
5. 1 tsp smoked paprika
6. 1 tsp ground chili
7. 1 tsp dried oregano
8. 1 tbsp. dried coriander
9. 400g chopped tomatoes

Instructions:

1. Heat some oil in a pan and fry the garlic and onion.
2. Add the ground beef and stir.
3. Add the spices, herbs, and tomatoes.
4. Simmer and stir while you make the avocado salsa, crepes, and vegetables.

Bacon and Beef Roll-Ups

Makes: 8 servings

Serving size: 1 cup

Calories: 345

Preparation time: 5 minutes

Nutritional information:

Fat   24g

Protein   28g

Carbohydrate   2g

Ingredients:

1. 4 slices streaky bacon
2. 4 steaks beef schnitzel
3. Handful spinach cheese

Instructions:

1. Place the beef schnitzel on your chopping board. Do same with the streaky bacon
2. .Place leafy greens on the streaky bacon.
3. Add cheese to the meat.
4. Roll the beef and fillings up.
5. Place each bacon roll and beef up in a baking tray.
6. Spray with oil.
7. Cook at 180C for 15 -20 minutes.

Malaysian Beef Curry

Makes: 6 servings

Serving size: 1 cup

Calories: 256

Preparation time: 10 minutes

Nutritional information:

Fat   14.1g

Protein   29.1g

Carbohydrate   2g

Ingredients:

1. 250 ml coconut cream
2. 800 g beef
3. 1 red onion
4. 1 tsp ground cardamom
5. 1/2 tsp chili powder
6. 1 tsp Chinese 5 spice
7. 1 tsp turmeric
8. 1 tsp ground cinnamon
9. 2 tsp cilantro ground
10. 1 tsp ground cumin
11. 4 cloves leafy greens

Instructions:

1. Place the coconut cream as well as other spices into a slow cooker and mix.
2. Add chopped beef and chopped onion, mix.
3. Cook mixture on low for about 8 - 10 hours.
5. Add leafy greens 5 minutes before serving.
6. Fold gently

Homemade Beef Jerky

Makes: 4 servings

Serving size: 100g

Calories: 320

Preparation time: 10 minutes

Nutritional information:

Fat   20g

Protein   35g

Carbohydrate   0g

Ingredients:

1. Extra virgin olive oil
2. Beef
3. Salt and pepper
4. Herbs Spices

Instructions:

1. Cut the beef into strips, 1-2cm wide.
2. Put the strips in a bowl with flavorings, and olive oil for coating the beef.
3. Mix the beef until coated with the flavor and oil.
4. Spread beef strips on your baking sheet.
5. Bake at 80C for 1 hour.
6. Turn the jerky beef strip over and bake/dehydrate for 30 minutes.

Fish Curry with Coconut and Spinach

Makes: 4 servings

Serving size: 100g

Calories: 314

Preparation time: 5 min

Nutritional information:

Fat   18.5g

Protein   33.4g

Carbohydrates 5.8g

Ingredients

1. 400 ml coconut cream
2. 1 kg white fish
3. 2-4 tbsp. curry paste
4. 400 ml coconut cream
5. 500 g spinach
6. 400 ml water

Instructions:

1. Heat oil in your saucepan, add curry paste and then fry on moderate heat for about 2-3 minutes.
2. Add the water and coconut cream and boil.
3. Add the fish pieces, reduce the heat and for 10-15 minutes.
4. Pour the prepared spinach. Cook for 3-4 minutes.

Meatloaf Cupcakes

Makes: 6 servings

Serving size: 1 cupcake

Calories: 221

Preparation time: 10 minutes

Nutritional information:

Fat 17.2g

Protein 15.2g

Carbohydrate 1g

Ingredients:

1. 2 eggs lightly beaten
2. Salt and pepper
3. 1 onion diced finely
4. 700g ground beef
5. 100g grated cheese

Instructions:

1. Mix the meat, diced onion, eggs, pepper, and salt.
2. Add flavoring and seasoning.
3. Mix all the ingredients with your hands and put a handful of meatloaf mixture into small muffin trays.
4. Cover with grated cheese, and sprinkle grated parmesan.
5. Cook at 180C/350F.

Parmesan-Encrusted Halibut

Makes: 6 servings

Serving size: 6 oz. per serving

Calories: 455

Preparation time: 5 minutes

Nutritional information:

Fat   30g

Protein   13g

Carbohydrates   2g

Ingredients:
1. 1 stick butter
2. 1-2 pounds halibut
3. 3 tsp grated Parmesan
4. 1 tsp kosher salt
5. 1 tsp panko breadcrumbs
6. 2 tsp garlic powder
7. ½ tsp black pepper
8. 1 tsp dried parsley

Instructions:
1. Pre-heat your oven to 400 degrees.
2. Blend all ingredients except the halibut.
3. Pat the halibut dry and lay each piece on a greased baking sheet.
4. Divide your Parmesan butter according to the number of fish you have.
5. Cook fish for about 10-12 minutes. Turn your broiler on high for approximately 2-3 minutes

Lamb meatballs

Makes: 24 meatballs

Serving size: 4 meatballs

Calories: 306

Preparation time: 20 minutes

Nutritional information:

Fat 17g

Protein   35g

Carbohydrates   2g

Ingredients:

Meatballs:

1. 2 eggs
2. 2 lbs. ground lamb
3. 1 clove garlic
4. 1/2 cup almond flour
5. 1/4 cup fresh parsley
6. 1 1/2 Tbsp. seasoning
7. 3 Tbsp. water
8. 1 tsp kosher salt
9. 2 Tbsp. olive oil

For the gremolata:

1. 1 Tbsp. lime zest
2. 2 Tbsp. fresh parsley
3. 2 cloves garlic
4. 2 Tbsp. chopped fresh mint

Instructions:

Meatballs:

1. Mix the meatball ingredients in a bowl and mix.

2. Mold into 24 1/2-inch meatballs.

3. Heat your olive oil in a sauté pan.

4. Cook your meatballs in batches.

5. Remove the cooked meatballs and put on a plate lined with paper towel until ready to serve.

Gremolata:

1. Mix the ingredients and mix well.

Keto teriyaki beef

Makes: 4 servings

Serving size: 4 oz. portion

Calories: 234

Preparation time: 20 minutes

Nutritional information:

Fat   9g

Protein   36g

Carbohydrate   5g

Ingredients:

1. 1 tsp sesame oil
2. 1 lb. lean beef
3. 1 tsp avocado oil
4. 2 Tbsp. soy sauce
5. 2 Tbsp. rice wine vinegar
6. 2 Tbsp. of erythritol granulated sweetener

Instructions:

1. Mix the avocado oil, sesame oil, soy sauce, sweetener and rice wine vinegar, in a medium bowl.
2. Place the beef pieces inside and stir.
3. Marinate for one hour or more.
4. Remove the beef from fridge 30 minutes.
5. Preheat the grill.
6. Divide the meat into four portions and thread onto four skewers with pieces of onion.
7. Grill beef skewers until it is ready
8. Cook the marinade in the microwave for about 2 minutes until cooked. Pour the sauce over skewers and serve

Keto buffalo chicken soup

Makes: 4 servings

Serving size: 100g

Calories: 406

Preparation time: 5 minutes

Nutritional information:

Fat   27g

Protein   29g

 Carbohydrate   5g

Ingredients:

1. 3 Tbsp. butter
2. 2 cups cooked chicken
3. 4 oz. cream cheese
4. 4 cups chicken broth
5. 1/3 cup Red Hot Sauce
6. Pepper and salt
7. ½ cup of Half and Half

Instructions:

1. Mix the butter, cream cheese, Half and Half, hot sauce, and chicken stock, in a blender and blend until smooth.
2. Take it to the small saucepan and cook for a while
3. Before serving, add the celery, shredded chicken, and blue cheese.

Sriracha Ranch Chicken

Makes: 4 servings

Serving size: 6 oz.

Calories: 129.9

Preparation time: 20 minutes

Nutritional information:

Fat 13g

Protein 1g

Carbohydrates 3g

Ingredients:

1. 1 tsp salt
2. 1/2 cup olive oil
3. 2-3 Tbsp. Sriracha
4. 1/2 cup ranch dressing
5. 1 tsp lemon juice
6. 3 Tbsp. Worcestershire sauce
7. 1 tsp white vinegar
8. 1 Tbsp. white sugar
9. 1/4 tsp black pepper
10. boneless, skinless chicken breast halves

Instructions:

1. Mix the olive oil, the Worcestershire sauce, ranch dressing, Sriracha, salt, white vinegar, lemon juice, pepper, and sugar.

2. Puree chicken breast

3. Place chicken in gallon-size ziplock bag,

4. Place the marinade over chicken.

5. Stir to coat.

6. Cover and refrigerate for 8 hours

7. Preheat the grill. Grill chicken for about 8 to 12 minute

Taco Lime Grilled Chicken

Makes: 4 servings

Serving size: 100g

Calories: 153

Preparation time: 5 minutes

Nutritional information:

Fat   2g

Protein   25g

Carbohydrate 3g

Ingredients:

1. 1/4 cup lime juice
2. 2 tablespoons taco seasoning
3. 1 pound skinless and boneless chicken breasts

Instructions:

1. Combine the lime juice and taco seasoning.
2. Cover the chicken breast inside the mixture and marinate for 30 minutes.
3. Grill on medium-high heat until it is cooked through.

Chicken and Avocado Burritos

Makes: 4 servings

Serving size: 100g

Calories: 519

Preparation time: 15 minutes

Nutritional information:

Fat   24g

Protein   40g

Carbohydrate   37.2g

Ingredients:

1. 1 large avocado
2. 4 burrito sized tortillas
3. 1 pound cooked chicken
4. 1 cup of Monterey Jack cheese
5. 1/4 cup salsa verde
6. 2 tablespoons cilantro
7. 1/4 cup sour cream

Instructions:

1. Assemble the burritos and enjoy!

Chicken in Creamy Parmesan with Sundried Tomato Sauce

Makes: 4 servings

Serving size: 6 oz.

Calories: 326

Preparation time: 30 minutes

Nutritional information:

Fat   12.8g

Protein   55.5g

Carbohydrates 2g

Ingredients:

1. 1 tablespoon oil
2. 2 cloves garlic
3. 4 boneless and skinless chicken breasts
4. 1/4 tsp red pepper flakes
5. 3/4 cup chicken broth
6. 1/4 cup white wine
7. 1/4 cup sundried tomatoes
8. 1/2 cup heavy/whipping cream
9. 1/4 cup parmesan, grated
10. 1/4 cup fresh basil
11. Salt and pepper

Instructions:

1. Heat your pan over medium-high heat.
2. Put the chicken and cook for 5 minutes per side.
3. Add the red pepper flakes, garlic, and sauté until fragrant
4. Add wine and deglaze your pan
5. Add cream, broth, sun-dried tomatoes as well as parmesan.
6. Boil on reduced heat. Simmer until sauce thickens for 3-5 minutes.
7. Add the chicken and any juices, season, and remove from heat.
8. Add the basil.

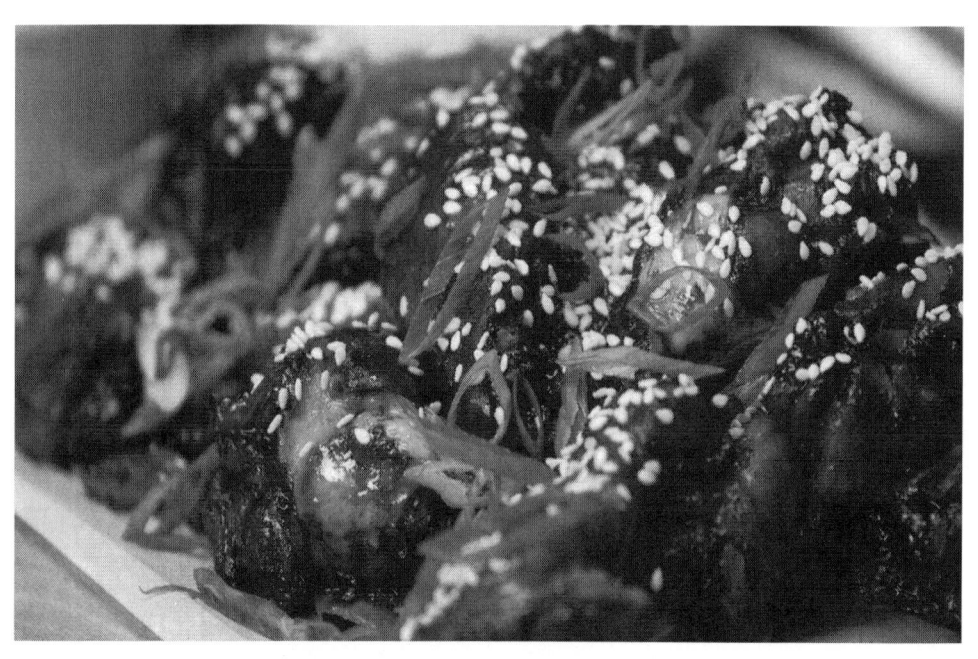

Dinner recipes

Spaghetti A la Carbonara

Makes: 4 servings

Serving size: 1 cup

Calories: 361

Preparation time: 20 minutes

Nutritional information:

Fat   28.84g

Protein   16.4g

Carbohydrates   4.67g

Ingredients:

1. 3 large eggs
2. 5 ounces bacon
3. 1 ½ tablespoons butter
4. 3 packages shirataki noodles
5. 2 large garlic cloves
6. 1 cup Parmesan cheese
7. Salt, parsley, and pepper.

Instructions:

1. Melt butter in pan.
2. Add bacon and cook until crispy.
3. Add minced garlic and shirataki noodles and turn down to medium-low.
4. Simmer.
5. Beat eggs and cheese (¾).
6. When noodles are warm, take it off and place in a separate bowl.
7. Stir in the egg/cheese mixture.
8. Top with parsley.

One Pot Shrimp Alfredo

Makes: 4 servings

Serving size: 1 cup

Calories: 297.83

Preparation time: 30 minutes

Nutritional information:

Fat   17.55g

Protein   22.93g

Carbohydrate   6.51g

Ingredients:

1. 1 pound raw shrimp
2. 1 tablespoon salted butter
3. 4 ounces cream cheese
4. 1 tablespoon garlic powder
5. ½ cup whole milk
6. 1 teaspoon salt
7. 1 teaspoon dried basil
8. 5 sun-dried tomatoes
9. ½ cup Parmesan cheese
10. ¼ cup baby kale

Instructions:

1. Melt the butter over medium heat.
2. Pour the shrimp into the skillet. Reduce the heat to medium low.
3. Cook both sides of your shrimp for 30 seconds.
4. Add cream cheese to the shrimp pan.
5. Add milk to the pan and increase the heat to medium.
6. Sprinkle the basil, garlic, and salt and stir.
7. Add the Parmesan cheese. Let simmer.
8. Fold sun-dried tomatoes as well as spinach or baby kale.

Keto Cordon Bleu

Makes: 7 servings

Serving size: 1 cup

Calories: 501.57

Preparation time: 20 minutes

Nutritional information:

Fat 35.65g

Protein 40.23g

Carbohydrates 1.45g

Ingredients:

1. 2 ounces pork rinds
2. Crumb Topping
3. 1/4 cup flaxseed meal
4. 1/2 teaspoon salt
5. 1/2 cup Parmesan cheese
6. 1/2 teaspoon garlic powder

Casserole Ingredients:

1. 2.3 pounds chicken breasts
2. Salt and black pepper
3. 8 slices ham
4. 8 slices Swiss cheese
5. 3 tablespoons butter

Sauce ingredients:

1. 2 tablespoons Dijon mustard
2. 3/4 cup mayonnaise

Instructions:

1. Heat oven to 350°F.
2. Blend flaxseed meal, pork rinds, garlic, Parmesan cheese, and 1/2 tsp of salt.
3. Cut the chicken breast and make six pieces.
4. Place the chicken in a casserole dish. Season with pepper and salt.
5. Place the ham on the chicken.
6. Place the Swiss cheese on the ham.
7. Layer the pork rind mix over the casserole.
8. Bake the casserole bare at 350°F for about 40-45 minutes.

Savory Italian Egg Bake

Makes: 8 servings

Serving size: 1 cup

Calories: 307

Preparation time: 20 minutes

Nutritional information: Fat 12.13g

Protein 13.3g

Carbohydrates 2.35g

Ingredients:

1. 10 large eggs
2. 2 teaspoons herb seasoning and garlic
3. 3 tablespoons mustard
4. ½ cup tomato sauce
5. ½ cup whipping cream
6. 12 ounces of frozen broccoli florets
7. 2 cups of diced cooked chicken breast
8. 1 teaspoon parsley flakes
9. ½ cup of grated Parmesan cheese
10. 1 cup of shredded sharp cheese

Instructions:

1. Preheat your oven to 350°F. Whisk the eggs.
2. Add the garlic, mustard, and herb seasoning, as well and heavy whipping cream.
3. Whisk the tomato sauce. Add the broccoli florets and diced chicken.
4. Grease your casserole dish then pour the Italian bake.
5. Add parsley flakes and Parmesan cheese on the Italian bake. Bake it for 30-40 minutes.
6. Top with extra sharp cheese.

Keto Sushi

Makes: 3 servings
Serving size: 1 1/2 rolls
Calories: 353
Preparation time: 5 minutes

Nutritional information:

Fat   25.7g
Protein   18.3g
Carbohydrates   5.7g

Ingredients:

1. 6 oz. Cream Cheese
2. 16 oz. Cauliflower
3. 1-2 tbsp. Rice Vinegar
4. 1 tbsp. Soy Sauce
5. 5 sheets Nori
6. 1/2 medium Avocado
7. 1 6-inch Cucumber
8. 5 oz. Smoked Salmon

Instructions:

1. Blend the cauliflower into small pieces by pulsing.
2. Cut the cucumber ends and slice off each side. Remove the middle and slice 2 sidepieces into tiny strips.
3. In a hot pan, add the cauliflower rice and cook. Add soy sauce.
4. Add the mix to a bowl with rice vinegar and cream cheese. Mix and set in the fridge.
5. Slice 1/2 avocado into tiny strips and scoop from the shell.
6. Place a nori sheet on a bamboo roller. Spread some cauliflower rice mixture over the sheet, add the fillings and roll tightly.

Keto Hot Chili Soup

Makes: 4 servings

Serving size: 1 cup

Calories: 369.5

Preparation time: 10 minutes

Nutritional information:

Fat   25.86g

Protein   27.03g

Carbohydrates 6.44g

Ingredients:

1. 2 tablespoons olive oil
2. 1 teaspoon coriander seeds
3. 2 cups chicken broth
4. 2 medium chili peppers
5. 2 cups water
6. ½ teaspoon ground cumin
7. 1 teaspoon turmeric
8. 16 ounces chicken thighs
9. 4 tablespoons tomato paste
10. 1 medium avocado
11. 2 tablespoons butter
12. 4 tbsp. chopped fresh cilantro
13. 2 ounces queso fresco
14. Salt and pepper
15. Juice of 1/2 lime

Instructions

1. Slice and set the chicken thighs and cook in an oiled pan.

2. In olive oil, heat the coriander seeds. Once heated, add in chili to season your oil.

3. Pour the water and broth and let it simmer. Season with ground cumin, turmeric, salt, and pepper.

4. Add your butter and tomato paste and stir.

5. Add the lime juice.

6. Put 4 ounces of chicken into bowls and ladle your soup. Garnish with avocado into, queso fresco and cilantro.

Keto Pumpkin Carbonara

Makes: 3 servings

Serving size: 4 oz.

Calories: 384

Preparation time: 20 minutes

Nutritional information:

Fat   34.7g

Protein 14g

Carbohydrates 2g

Ingredients:

1. 5 oz. Pancetta
2. 1 package Shirataki Noodles
3. 1/4 cup Heavy Cream
4. 2 large Egg Yolks
5. 2 tbsp. Butter
6. 1/3 cup Parmesan Cheese
7. 1/2 tsp. Dried Sage
8. 3 tbsp. Pumpkin Puree
9. Salt and Pepper

Instructions:

1. Place shirataki noodles in hot water for 2 minutes.
2. Chop pancetta and pour into a hot pan.
3. Place butter in a small pot and allow it to get brown. Add the pumpkin puree and sage.
4. Add pancetta fat and heavy cream to the pan and mix.
5. Add the shirataki noodles.
6. Add the parmesan cheese and mix well.
7. Add pancetta and noodles into the sauce and turn well.
8. Add two egg yolks and mix.

Coconut Curry Chicken Tenders

Makes: 5 servings

Serving size: 4 oz.

Calories: 494

Preparation time: 30 minutes

Nutritional information:

Fat   39.4g

Protein   29.4g

Carbohydrates 2.1g

Ingredients:

1. 1 large Egg
2. Coconut Curry Chicken Tenders
3. 2 tsp. Curry Powder
4. 24 oz. Chicken Thighs
5. 1/2 cup Pork Rinds
6. 1/2 cup Shredded Coconut
7. 1/4 tsp. Garlic Powder
8. 1/4 tsp. Onion Powder
9. 1/2 tsp. Coriander
10. Salt and Pepper

Dipping Sauce:

1. 1/4 cup Sour Cream
2. 1/4 cup Mayonnaise
3. 1 1/2 tsp. Mango Extract
4. 2 tbsp. Sugar-Free Ketchup
5. 1/2 tsp. Garlic Powde

6. 1/2 tsp. Red Pepper Flakes
7. 1/4 tsp. Cayenne Pepper
8. 1/2 tsp. Ground Ginger
9. 7 drops Liquid Stevia

Instructions:

1. Pre-heat your oven to 400F.
2. Beat egg. Debone chicken with skin on, and cut chicken into thin strips.
3. Place coconut, pork rinds, and spices in a plastic bag. Add chicken and then shake.
4. Place the tenders on a wire rack. Bake for 15 minutes and flip each tender, and bake.
5. Combine the sauce ingredients and mix.

Chicken Pad Thai

Makes: 4 servings

Serving size: 6 oz.

Calories: 431

Preparation time: 10 minutes

Nutritional information:

Fat 35.3g

Protein   26.3g

Carbohydrates 5g

Ingredients:

1. Juice 1/2 Lime
2. Pad Thai Sauce
3. 1/2 tsp. Worcestershire Sauce
4. Juice 1/3 Lemon
5. 1 1/2 tbsp. Sambal Olek
6. 1 1/2 tbsp. Ketchup
7. 1 1/2 tsp. Minced Garlic
8. 3 tbsp. Fish Sauce
9. 1 tsp. Rice Wine Vinegar
10. 7 drops Liquid Stevia
11. 1 tbsp. Natural Peanut Butter

Noodles and Toppings ingredients:

1. 3 medium Green Onions
2. 1/4 cup Cilantro
3. 2 large Eggs
4. medium Chicken Thighs
5. 2 packets Shirataki Noodles
6. 4 oz. Mung Bean Sprouts
7. 4 tbsp. Coconut Oil
8. 2 tbsp. Peanuts

Instructions:

1. Blend the ingredients for your sauce with a whisk.
2. Drain the shirataki noodles and rinse. Repeat six times and dry.
3. Debone and deskin the chicken thighs, and slice.
4. Heat the Coconut Oil over medium-high heat. Add the chicken.
5. Add the shirataki noodles. Dry fry for 5-8 minutes. Add two eggs.
6. Add the chicken, sauce, cilantro, as well as green onion.

Low-Carb Chicken Curry

Makes: 3 servings

Serving size: 1 cup

Calories: 493

Preparation time: 30 minutes

Nutritional information:

Fat   35g

Protein   37.5g

Carbohydrates   4.8g

Ingredients:

1. 1 Green Chili
2. 2 tbsp. Coconut Oil
3. 2 Shallots
4. 1.5 inch Ginger
5. 2 cloves Garlic
6. 1 stalk Lemongrass
7. 2 tsp. Turmeric Powder
8. 1/2 cup Water
9. 1/2 cup Coconut Milk
10. 1/2 tsp. Salt
11. 21 oz. Chicken
12. 1 tbsp. chopped Cilantro

Instructions:

1. Cut Lemongrass.
2. Pound shallots, ginger, Green Chili, and garlic.

3. Sauté all pounded ingredients in your Coconut Oil over medium heat.

4. After about 3-4 minutes, add the turmeric powder and the sliced Lemongrass. Sauté again.

5. Add Chicken and mix.

6. Pour water and coconut milk and mix. Add Salt and stir.

7. Sprinkle Cilantro

Salmon with Tarragon Dill Cream Sauce

Makes: 2 servings

Serving size: 1 cup

Calories: 46

Preparation time: 30 minutes

Nutritional information:

Fat   40g

Protein   22.5g

Carbohydrates 1.5g

Ingredients:

1. 1 1/2 lb. Salmon Filet
2. 3/4-1 tsp. Dried Tarragon
3. 1 tbsp. Duck Fat
4. Salt and Pepper
5. 3/4-1 tsp. of Dried Dill Weed

Cream Sauce ingredients:

1. 2 tbsp. Butter
2. 1/2 tsp. Dried Tarragon
3. 1/4 cup Heavy Cream
4. 1/2 tsp. Dried Dill Weed
5. Pepper and Salt

Instructions:

1. Cut the salmon in half. Season fish with spices and salt and pepper.

2. Heat the duck fat in ceramic cast iron skillet. Add the salmon skin side down.

3. Let the salmon cook while skin crisps up.////////

4. Cook the salmon. 7-15 minutes on low heat.

5. Remove it from the pan. Add spices and butter to the pan. Once browned, add the cream mix.

Orange and Sage Glazed Duck Breast

Makes: 1 serving

Serving size: 100g

Calories: 798

Preparation time: 30 minutes

Nutritional information:

Fat   71g

Protein   36g

Carbohydrate 0g

Ingredients:

1. 1/4 tsp. Sage
2. 1 6 oz. Duck Breast
3. 1 tbsp. Heavy Cream
4. 2 tbsp. Butter
5. 1/2 tsp. Orange Extract
6. 1 tbsp. Sweetener
7. 1 cup Spinach

Instructions:

1. Season duck breast with salt and pepper.
2. Add butter and swerve in the pan.
3. Add orange extract and sage.
4. Put the duck breast in a cold pan and set to medium-high.
5. Flip the duck.
6. Add the heavy cream to the sauce, and then stir. Pour it over the duck in the pan and mix with duck fat. Cook the mix.
7. Add some spinach in the pan.

Perfect Ribeye Steak

Makes: 2 servings

Serving size: 1 cup

Calories: 750

Preparation time: 30 minutes

Nutritional information:

Fat 66g

Protein 38g

Carbohydrates 0g

Ingredients:

1. 1 tbsp. Butter
2. 1 16 oz. Ribeye Steak
3. 1 tbsp. Duck Fat
4. 1/2 tsp. Thyme
5. Salt and Pepper

Instructions:

1. Preheat the oven to 400F. Prepare the steak by seasoning with salt, oil, and pepper.
2. Remove the pan from oven when pre-heated and place on the stove. Add the oil and steak to the pan. Allow to sear for 2 minutes.
3. Flip the steak and put it in the oven for 6 minutes. Remove the steak. Place over low heat.
4. Add thyme and butter into the pan and moisten steak for 4 minutes.
5. Allow to rest for 5 minutes.

Roasted Red Bell Pepper and Cauliflower Soup

Makes: 5 servings

Serving size: 1 cup

Calories: 345

Preparation time: 20 minutes

Nutritional information:

Fats   32g

Protein   6.4g

Carbohydrates   6.2g

Ingredients:

1. 6 tbsp. Duck Fat
2. 2 small Red Bell Peppers
3. 1/2 head Cauliflower
4. 3 medium Green Onions
5. 3 cups Chicken Broth
6. 1/2 cup Heavy Cream
7. 1 tsp. Dried Thyme
8. 1 tsp. Garlic Powder
9. 1/4 tsp. of Red Pepper Flakes
10. 1 tsp. Smoked Paprika
11. 4 oz. Goat Cheese
12. Salt and Pepper

Instructions:

1. Slice the peppers in half. De-seed them. Pound for 15 minutes or until the skin is blackened.

2. Cut cauliflower into tiny florets and season with melted duck fat, pepper, and salt. Roast cauliflower in the oven for 35 minutes.

3. Remove the skin from the peppers.

4. In a pot, bring four tbsp. of duck fat and heat it with add cubed green onion. Add the seasoning to toast, and add red pepper, chicken broth, and cauliflower. Let simmer for 20 minutes.

5. Use an immersion blender. Add cream and mix.

6. Garnish with green onion and extra thyme.

Bacon Cheeseburger Soup

Makes: 5 servings

Serving size: 1 cup

Calories: 572

Preparation time: 30 minutes

Nutritional information:

Fat   48.6g

Protein   23.4g

Carbohydrates 3.4g

Ingredients:

1. 2 tbsp. Butter
2. 3 cups Beef Broth
3. 5 slices Bacon
4. 1/2 tsp. Garlic Powder
5. 12 oz. Ground Beef
6. 1/2 tsp. Onion Powder
7. 1 1/2 tsp. Kosher Salt
8. 2 tsp. Brown Mustard
9. 1/2 tsp. Red Pepper
10. 1/2 tsp. Black Pepper
11. 1 tsp. Chili Powder
12. 1 tsp. Cumin
13. 1 medium Dill Pickle
14. 2 1/2 tbsp. Tomato Paste
15. 1 cup Cheddar Cheese
16. 1/2 cup Heavy Cream
17. 3 oz. Cream Cheese

Instructions:

1. Cook the bacon in a pan until crispy.
2. Add the ground beef, cook until brown, and flip the other side.
3. Take the beef to the pot. Add spices and butter to the pan let it stay for 30-45 seconds.
4. Add the tomato paste, beef broth, mustard, pickles, and cheese and let cook until melted.
5. Cover the pot and turn it to low heat. Let cook for 20-30 minutes.
6. Turn off the stove; finish with crumbled bacon and heavy cream. Stir well.

Snacks recipe

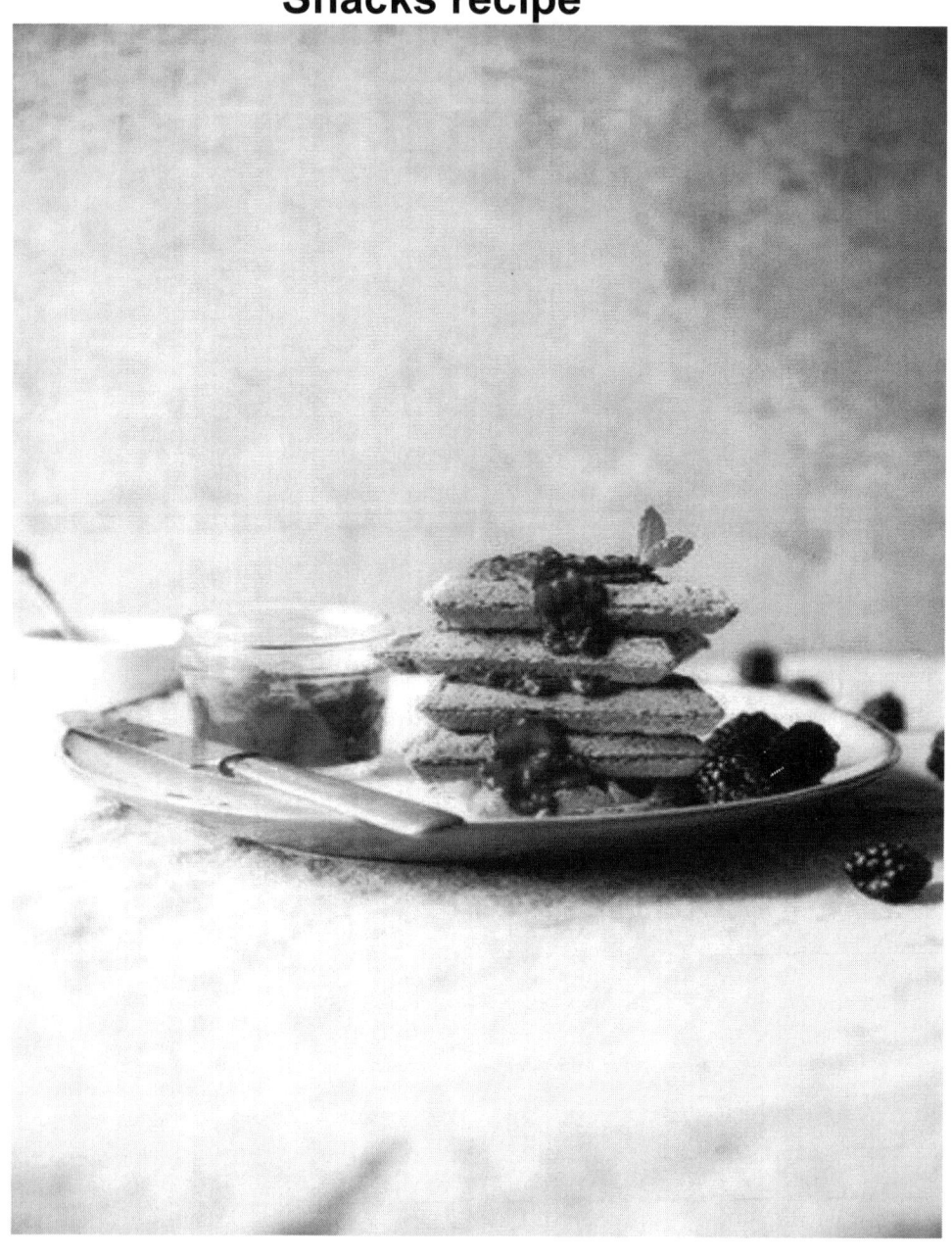

Almonds Italiano

Makes: 3 servings Serving size: 1/4-cup

Makes: 1 serving

Calories: 277

Preparation time: 30 minutes

Nutritional information:

Fat   25g

Protein   9g

Carbohydrate   10g

Ingredients:

1. 1 egg white
2. 2 tablespoons olive oil
3. 2 teaspoons garlic powder
4. 8 teaspoons Italian seasoning
5. 1/2 teaspoon salt
6. 2 teaspoons onion powder
7. 3 cups unblanched almonds

Instructions:

1. Whisk the egg white, oil, spices, and salt.
2. Add nuts mixing well to coat the almonds.
3. Spread evenly in a single layer.
4. Then bake at 275° for 45 minutes. Stir every 10 minutes.

TortillaChips

Serving size: 9 wraps

Calories: 161

Preparation time: 20 minutes

Nutritional information:

Fat   13g

Protein   9g

Carbohydrate   3g

Ingredients:

1. 1 Sherrielee's Tortilla Wrap

Instructions:

1. Slice the tortilla wrap into 6 wedges.
2. Place on your microwave-safe dinner plate.
3. Microwave on high for 1 minute.
4. Watch closely so they do not burn.

Almond Flour Crisps

Makes: 1 serving

Serving size: 8 crackers

Calories: 212

Preparation time: 5 minutes

Nutritional information:

Fat   16g

Protein 15g

Carbohydrates 4g

Ingredients:

1. Salt
2. 1/4 cup grated parmesan cheese
3. 2 tbsp. almond flour

Instructions:

1. Line the baking sheet with a silicone liner.
2. Mix the ingredients and put them in eight mounds on the baking sheet.
3. Flatten each mound with your finger.
4. Bake at 400° for six minutes. Do not microwave.

Microwave Flax Crackers

Makes: 1 serving

Serving size: 1 cup

Calories: 137

Preparation time: 5 minutes

Nutritional information:

Fat 11g

Protein   7g

Carbohydrates 7g

Ingredients:

1. 1 tsp sesame seeds
2. 2 tsp flax meal
3. 1 tsp parmesan cheese
4. 1/2 tsp Seasoning Salt
5. 1 tsp water

Instructions:

1. Mix the ingredients in a bowl until the dough forms.
2. Use parchment paper and shape the dough into about 6-8 thin circles.
3. Place the parchment in the microwave and cook for 1 minutes

WPI Crackers

Makes: 12 servings

Serving size: 12 crackers

Calories: 287

Preparation time: 5 minutes

Nutritional information:

Fat   24g

Protein   16g

Carbohydrate   2g

Ingredients:

1. 1/2 cup butter
2. 8 ounces cheddar cheese
3. 1 cup of wheat protein isolate
4. 1/2 cup almond flour
5. 1/2 teaspoon salt

Instructions:

1. Put the butter and cheese in a food processor.
2. Process for 1-2 minutes until creamy, scraping the sides.
3. Add the ingredients and process.
4. Using some cookie scoop, and drop the dough on a parchment baking sheet.
5. Cover the balls with a plastic wrap and take the baking powder can, and press down on each ball of dough.
6. Remove the plastic wrap until the wafers are shaped.
7. Bake for 11-12 minutes.
8. Remove from pan and set on a cooling rack.

Chewy Peanut Butter Candy

Makes: 4-8 servings

Serving size: 1 bar

Calories: 107

Preparation time: 5 minutes

Nutritional information:

Fat 7g

Protein   9g

Carbohydrate   2g

Ingredients:

1. 1/4 cup peanut butter
2. 2 tablespoons butter
3. 1 cup of chocolate whey protein powder
4. 1/4 cup liquid Splenda
5. 1/4 cup of Da Vinci syrup

Instructions:

1. Melt your butter in the microwave.
2. Add the peanut butter until smooth and stir in your Splenda.
3. Add protein powder and mix.
4. Add the syrup until you have a glossy, caramel-like goo.
5. Put this into a tiny non-stick container and freeze.

Chocolate Almond Bar

Makes: 2 servings

Serving size: 1 bar

Calories: 33

Preparation time: 5 minutes

Nutritional information:

Fat 3g

Protein   1g

Carbohydrate 1g

Ingredients:

1. 2 tablespoons butter
2. 1/2 ounce unsweetened chocolate
3. 1 teaspoon cream
4. 1-ounce almonds
5. 4 teaspoons granular Splenda
6. 1/8 teaspoon vanilla
7. 2 ounces almonds
8. 1/8 teaspoon almond extract

Instructions:

1. Melt the butter and chocolate in the microwave.
2. Blend well. Add the ingredients.
3. Spread into a thick rectangle on the foil-lined pan and freeze for 2 hours.
4. Remove from the foil, slice into 40-48 pieces.

Chocolate Coconut Bark

Makes: 4 servings

Serving size: 1 bar

Calories: 145

Preparation time: 5 minutes

Nutritional information:

Fat   16g

Protein   1g

Carbohydrate 1g

Ingredients:

1. 1/4 cup coconut oil
2. 20 grams cocoa chocolate
3. 1 tsp granular Splenda

Instructions:

1. Break the chocolate into small pieces.
2. Put it in a microwaveable bowl with your coconut oil.
3. Microwave for 1 minute and add the Splenda.
4. Stir to blend. Pour into a container that is lined with nonstick foil.
5. Store in freezer until firm. Break into pieces.

Coconut Fudge

Makes: 4 servings

Serving size: 1 bar

Calories: 183

Preparation time: 5 minutes

Nutritional information:

Fat   18g

Protein   3g

Carbohydrate   6g

Ingredients:

1. 2 tablespoons cocoa
2. 1/4 cup of virgin coconut oil
3. 1/2-1 cup of granular Splenda
4. 2 tbsp. natural peanut butter

Instructions:

1. In a bowl, microwave your coconut oil.
2. Whisk the peanut butter and the cocoa. Add it to the mix.
3. Add Splenda and pour into a non-stick foil-lined container. Freeze until solid, 20- 30 minutes.
4. Cut into squares using a sharp knife.

Whey Protein Not Cake

Makes: 6 serving

Serving size: 1 bar

Calories: 119

Preparation time: 5 minutes

Nutritional information:

Fat 9g

Protein   8g

Carbohydrate   2g

Ingredients:

1. 1 egg
2. 4 tablespoons butter
3. 1/2 cup whey protein powder
4. 1/4 cup granular Splenda

Instructions:

1. Measure and melt the butter in the microwave.
2. Pour the Splenda and mix.
3. Add the egg and protein powder.
4. Mix well until it is smooth.
5. Pour it into the greased baking dish.
6. Bake for 8 minutes.
7. Cool and cut into squares.

Sauce recipes

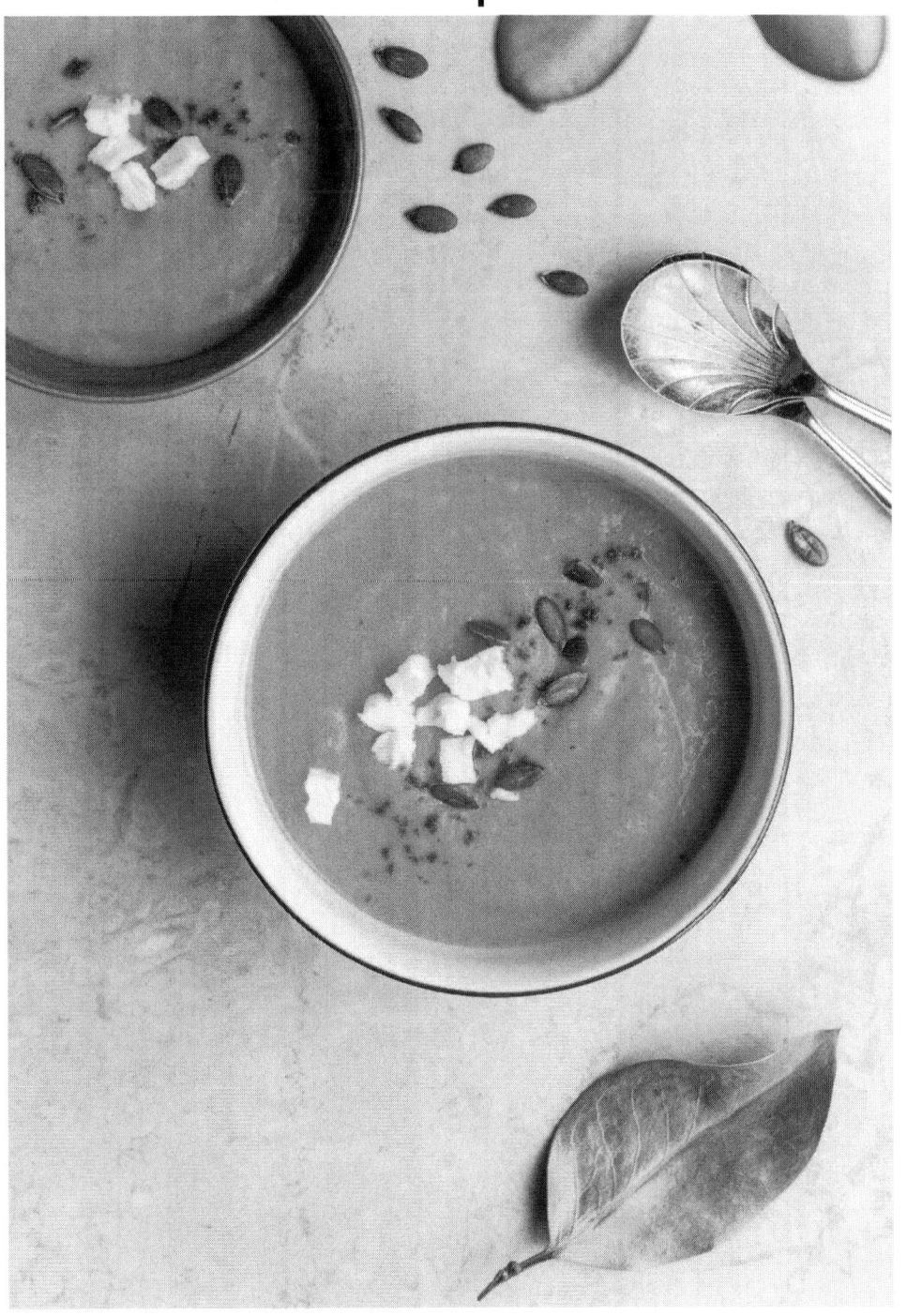

Brown Butter Cream sauce

Makes: 6 servings

Serving size: 1 cup

Calories: 100 calories

Preparation time: 5 minutes

Nutritional information:

Fat   3g

Protein 5g

Carbohydrates   2g

Ingredients:

1. 1 clove Garlic
2. 4 tbsp. Butter
3. 1/2 tsp Salt
4. 1/4 cup Chicken broth
5. 1/2 tsp Pepper
6. 1/3 cup Cream

Instructions:

1. Brown your butter in a pan over medium heat.
2. Add the brown butter and add chicken broth, garlic, cream, pepper, and salt.
3. Stir until combined
4. Reduce heat to simmer.
5. Stir lightly until the sauce thickens.

Keto Spicy BBQ Sauce

Makes: 10 Tsp

Serving size: 1 cup

Calories: 10.36
Preparation time: 10 servings

Nutritional information:

Fat   0.13g

Protein 0.54g

Carbohydrates   1.69g

Ingredients:

1. 6oz water
2. ¼ onion
3. 1 Tsp Coconut Oil
4. 1 Tbsp. Garlic
5. 1 6oz can Tomato Paste
6. 2 Tsp salt
7. ¼ cup yellow mustard
8. ½ Tbsp. Paprika
9. 1 Tbsp. Chili Powder
10. 1 Tsp Cumin
11. 1 Dash Tabasco Sauce
12. 1 Tsp Cayenne Pepper

Instructions:

1. Using a skillet, melt the coconut oil and sauté garlic and onion.
2. Add all other ingredients. Stir and let simmer.
3. Add water if it thickens
4. Use Cayenne along with Tabasco and 1 Tsp sweetener for a sweet sauce

Cocktail Sauce

Makes: 10 Tsp

Serving size: 1 cup

Calories: 6.3

Preparation time: 5 minutes

Nutritional information:

Fat   0.06g

Protein 0.39g

Carbohydrates   1.5g

Ingredients:

1. 2 tablespoons lemon juice
2. 1 cup of sugar-free ketchup
3. ¼ teaspoon of Frank's hot sauce
4. 1/3 cup prepared horseradish
5. ½ tablespoon of Worcestershire sauce

Instructions:

1. Place all ingredients in an emulsion blender container.
2. Blend until well combined,
3. Serve with seafood.

Enchilada Sauce

Makes: 6 servings

Serving size: 1 cup

Calories: 188

Preparation time: 5 minutes

Nutritional information:

Fat   18g

Protein   2g

Carbohydrates 8g

Ingredients:

1. 2 teaspoons Dried Oregano
2. 3 ounces Butter
3. 1/4 teaspoon Cayenne
4. 3 teaspoons Cumin
5. 2 teaspoons Coriander
6. 2 teaspoons Onion Powder
7. 1 1/2 tablespoons Erythritol
8. 12 ounces Tomato Puree
9. 1/2 teaspoon Salt
10. 1/2 teaspoon Pepper

Instructions:

1. Place butter in a saucepan on the stove over medium heat.
2. Add all the ingredients except your tomato puree. Sauté for about 3 minutes.
3. Add your tomato puree and stir.
5. Simmer for 5 minutes. Add some water and adjust the seasoning as desired.

Sweet Soy Sauce

Makes: 16 servings

Serving size: 1 cup

Calories: 8

Preparation time: 5 minutes

Nutritional information:

Fat   0g

Protein   2g

Carbohydrates 1g

Ingredients:

1. 1 ¼ cup Erythritol
2. 8 ounces Tamari Sauce

Instructions:

1. Put the ingredients in your saucepan over low heat.
2. Dissolve the erythritol and heat for 15-20 minutes.

Grocery list

Avocado

Apples

Apricot

Blueberries

Bananas

Blackberries

Cherries

Cranberries

Dates

Figs

Grapefruit

Grapes

Guava

Kiwi

Limes

Lemons

Mango

Melons

Nectarines

Oranges

Olives

Pears

Papaya

Passion Fruit

Peaches

Pineapples

Pomegranates

Plums

Raspberry

Rhubarb

Strawberries

Tomatoes

Tangerines

Sour Cream

Heavy Whipping Cream

Mayonnaise

Full Cream Greek Yogurt

Full Cream Milk

Cheeses:

Blue

Brie

Cottage Cheese

Cheddar

Colby

Cream Cheese

Feta

Goat Cheese

Mozzarella

Monterey Jack

Parmesan

Swiss

String Cheeses

Hamburger

Roast Beef

Steak

Corned Beef

Prime Rib

Baby Back Ribs

Pork:

Ham

Bacon

Pork Roast

Tenderloin

Pork Chops

Ground Pork

Sausages:

Italian Sausage

Deli Ham

Hot Dogs

Lamb

Pepperoni

Canned Chicken:

Chicken Legs

Chicken Breasts

Chicken Thighs

Chicken Tenders

Whole Chicken

Chicken Wings

Cornish Hens

Chicken Eggs

Fish:

Catfish

Cod

Crab

Haddock

Flounder

Halibut

Herring

Oysters

Lobster

Salmon

Sardines

THANK YOU FOR BUYING MY BOOK!

Just take your gift from me

http://www.bestsellers.pp.ua/robertstill/

Thank You!

Robert Still

Diet plan

	Breakfast	Snack	Lunch	Snack	Dinner
Monday	Three scrambled eggs. 1 100% meat sausage. Two rashers bacon	Devilled eggs	Spicy chicken, mixed leaf, spinach, and bacon salad	Mixed nuts. Natural yoghurt	Wilted spinach, Fried salmon fillet Toasted almonds
Tuesday	Mixed pepper, spinach omelet/ frittata	Mixed seeds/smooth almond nut butter	Egg with bacon muffin cups	Cottage cheese	Coconut shrimps with mixed veggies
Wednesday	Cheese and bacon omelet	Mixed nuts and Natural yogurt	Ham and cheese roll-ups served with wilted spinach	½ ripe avocado	Spicy chicken wings
Thursday	Smoked salmon, Poached eggs, sliced avocado	Natural peanut butter and mixed seeds	Mayonnaise salad, Basic tuna with romaine lettuce	Cheese strings	Roasted bell peppers, Spicy minced beef Mozzarella cheese
Friday	Sugar-free syrup, Low-carb protein pancakes, Crispy bacon	Boiled eggs	Spicy minced beef	Mixed nut and String cheese	Baked spicy chicken thighs, Cheesy cauliflower, broccoli puree, Handful of mixed nuts

Why you should keep track of your figure and health

Keeping track of your health and figure goes beyond staying trim. It could go a long way to improve your body image and show you how many calories you're consuming daily. When you keep track of your nutrition, you will be able to tell if you are eating enough fruits, vegetables, and whole grains. All of which are essential for optimum health. Tracking solid fats, desserts, and oils will enable you to determine if you are consuming these foods excessively.

Your body image encompasses your feelings about your physical appearance. If you want to change certain things about your body, you can meet a dietician to help you reach your body goals. As a rule, ensure that the goals you set are realistic for the kind of body you have. Tracking the progress you have made and achieving these goals will boost your self-esteem as well as your body image.

Another crucial reason to keep track of your figure is that not eating properly leads to health risks. Several reports have shown that a third of adults in the US alone are obese. The number of overweight children is also increasing rapidly.

Following some of these simple recipes will improve your quality of life and keep you healthy and young.

All rights Reserved. No part of this publication or the information in it may be quoted from or reproduced in any form by means such as printing, scanning, photocopying or otherwise without prior written permission of the copyright holder.

Disclaimer and Terms of Use: Effort has been made to ensure that the information in this book is accurate and complete, however, the author and the publisher do not warrant the accuracy of the information, text and graphics contained within the book due to the rapidly changing nature of science, research, known and unknown facts and internet. The Author and the publisher do not hold any responsibility for errors, omissions or contrary interpretation of the subject matter herein. This book is presented solely for motivational and informational purposes only.

Printed in Great Britain
by Amazon